D0322539

H0701523   WE140

Updne 20/7/23

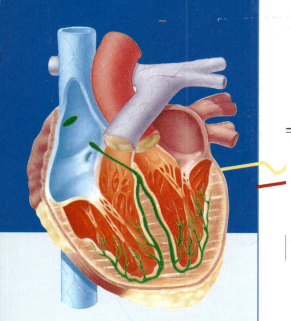

This book is due for return on or before the last date shown below.

- 4 FEB 2008

0 6 JUN 2008

25 OCT

08/01/18

- 6 NOV 2009

0 9 APR 2010

1 5 NOV 2010

0 3 AUG 2012

2 May 2013

- 3 DEC 2013

G

BRENDA M. BEASLEY
BS, RN, EMT-Paramedic

Croydon Health Sciences Library
Mayday University Hospital
London Road
Thornton Heath
Surrey CR7 7YE

Prentice Hall

Upper Saddle River, New Jersey 07458

Library of Congress Cataloging-in-Publication Data

Beasley, Brenda M.
   Understanding EKGs : a practical approach / Brenda Beasley.--2nd ed.
      p. cm.
   Includes index.
   ISBN 0-13-045215-7
      1. Electrocardiography. I. Title.

RC683.5.E5 B378 2003
616.1'207547--dc21   2002038107

Publisher: Julie Levin Alexander
Publisher's Assistant: Regina Bruno
Executive Editor: Marlene Pratt
Editorial Assistant: Monica Silva
Senior Managing Editor: Lois Berlowitz
Director of Production and Manufacturing: Bruce Johnson
Managing Production Editor: Patrick Walsh
Manufacturing Manager: Ilene Sanford
Manufacturing Buyer: Pat Brown
Production Liaison: Jeanne Molenaar
Production Editor: Emily Bush, Carlisle Communications, Inc.
Design Director: Cheryl Asherman
Design Coordinator: Christopher Weigand
Cover Designer: Blair Brown
Interior Designer: Janice Bielawa
Senior Marketing Manager: Katrin Beacom
Product Information Manager: Rachele Strober
Composition: Carlisle Communications, Inc.
Printing and Binding: Von Hoffman Press
Cover Printer: Coral Graphics

Pearson Education LTD.
Pearson Education Australia PTY, Limited
Pearson Education Singapore, Pte. Ltd
Pearson Education North Asia Ltd
Pearson Education Canada, Ltd
Pearson Educación de Mexico, S.A. de C.V.
Pearson Education—Japan
Pearson Education Malaysia, Pte. Ltd

Copyright © 2003 by Pearson Education, Inc., Upper Saddle River, New Jersey 07458. All rights reserved. Printed in the United States of America. This publication is protected by Copyright and permission should be obtained from the publisher prior to any prohibited reproduction, storage in a retrieval system, or transmission in any form or by any means, electronic, mechanical, photocopying, recording, or likewise. For information regarding permission(s), write to: Rights and Permissions Department.

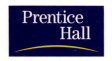

10 9 8 7 6
ISBN 0-13-045215-7

Dedication

This book is dedicated to a very special group of people who have always been the lights of my life: Ben, Stephanie, Cody, Landon, Corey, Logan, Ashton, Trey, Harper, Anna Caitlyn, and Mary Patton . . . my precious nieces and nephews . . . my inspiration.

and to

Michael C. West, MS, RN, EMT-P

Your assistance, support, encouragement, and constancy were invaluable to me throughout this revision process and I am very grateful for, and blessed by, your friendship.

Brief Contents

Contents

REVIEWERS

I wish to thank the following reviewers for providing invaluable feedback and suggestions during the revision of this text:

John L. Beckman
Firefighter/Paramedic
Affiliated with Addison Fire Protection District
Addison, Illinois
EMS Instructor
Deerfield, IL

Marilyn Ermish, NREMT-P
American Medical Response
Cheyenne, Wyoming

Jarrod Taylor, NREMT-P, RN, BSN
Calhoun Community College
Decatur, AL

Jim Williams, CCEMT-P, NREMT-P
Training Officer, Medical Center EMS
Bowling Green, KY

I also wish to thank the following professionals who reviewed the first edition of *Understanding EKGs: A Practical Approach*:

John L. Beckman
Firefighter/Paramedic
Affiliated with Addison Fire
Protection District
Addison, Illinois
EMS Instructor
Deerfield, IL

Benjamin J. Camp, MD
Emergency Medicine Physician
Tanner Medical Center
124 West Club Drive
Carrollton, GA

James M. Courtney, NREMT-P
Vermont Department of Health
Office of Emergency Services
Burlington, VT

Marilyn Ermish, NREMT-P
American Medical Response
Cheyenne, Wyoming

Willis D. Israel, MD
P.O. Box 129
Wedowee, AL

Willie King, RN, MSN, CNS
Nursing Instructor
Calhoun Community College
P.O. Box 2216
Decatur, AL

John A. Rasmussen, PhD, NREMT-P
Education Coordinator
Greenville County EMS
Greenville, SC

Jarrod Taylor, NREMT-P, RN
Calhoun Community College
Decatur, AL

Foreword

When advanced life-support training for paramedical personnel was still considered questionable by most of my physician colleagues, I became involved in teaching advanced cardiac life support (ACLS). It soon became apparent that emergency medical technicians—in those days very frequently volunteer and/or part-time workers in the field—were frequently the most enthusiastic and responsive students of ACLS. Their eagerness to learn and to provide the whole range of prehospital care has proved to be a huge factor in patient survival.

I loved every moment I taught ACLS (as well as BCLS, emergency medical technician training, and advanced trauma life support)—whether to physicians, nurses, or paramedical personnel. Indeed, the teachers of these basic and extremely important concepts have impacted all areas of current medical care. Many of those with whom I taught ACLS became my close and greatly cherished friends. One of these is Brenda Messer Beasley, BS, RN, EMT-P, with whom I shared in teaching the first EMT course ever offered in rural Randolph County, Alabama. From the initial class session, I saw that Ms. Beasley had an extraordinary ability to render a complicated concept in its most basic form of expression. Though she had this gift for rendering the complex in simple terms, she never allowed the importance of what she was teaching to be lost, and she always stressed the awareness of and evaluation of the patient.

Ms. Beasley brings to this text on EKG interpretation the same ability to simplify the complex for the health care professional. Real meaning is surely more valuable than the easy "information overload" encountered when we deal with real patients in a medical emergency.

After I had taught with Ms. Beasley, she made a career change from nursing to full-time EMT training, still in our same basic geographical area. It became fun and rewarding as a practicing small-town family physician to be aware of prehospital care that had been rendered by students of this teacher. Their expertise was (is) impressive, as was their attention to the care of and the state of the patient. Certainly, any physician's ability to treat, and any patient's ultimate well-being, depends greatly on that initial prehospital care.

An appropriate text on EKG interpretation can only deepen the perception and understanding of the health care professional; at the same time, this text seems to teach and reteach the basic concept from every situation: "First, look at your patient, and continue to look at your patient."

I am honored to welcome this book to the plentiful material available on the heart, its functions, the circulatory system and its signals of dysfunction and illness.

Willis D. Israel, M.D.
Wedowee, Alabama

Preface

This book represents an informative and simple approach to EKG analysis. Based on the fact that cardiology and basic EKG interpretation are integral parts of most primary and allied-health-related curricula, I wrote this book to assist the novice student in his/her understanding of basic EKG interpretation. This book is intended for the health care provider at the initial level(s) of understanding of cardiovascular anatomy, physiology, and rhythm strip interpretation. The categories of students who will benefit from this text include prehospital care providers, medical students, cardiac care monitor techs, ACLS candidates, nursing professionals, physician assistants, respiratory therapy students, and cardiac technology students.

This EKG book consists of fifteen chapters that are designed to provide the user with a practical, yet comprehensive, approach to the skill of EKG interpretation. The strategy of this manuscript has centered around producing a useful guide to the understanding of abnormal heart rhythms, ie., dysrhythmias, for the health care provider in his/her provision of optimum patient care. In order to afford the instructor and the student the opportunity to work in a reasonable order through the technical information, the material has been presented in such a manner as to achieve understanding of each chapter prior to proceeding to the next chapter. The content is presented in short, succinct chapters in order to facilitate comprehension of each concept in a "building block" format.

In this revised edition of the book, each chapter now contains a section of multiple choice items to be used for self-assessment and review. The book includes expanded graphics, as well as rhythm strip examples, review strips, and end-of-chapter questions to afford the student a comprehensive mastery of the material. Answers to review questions and review strips are provided in the appendix at the back of the book. Also included in this second edition of the book is a chapter dedicated to the assessment and management of the patient with cardiovascular emergencies. The term **dysrhythmia** is used throughout the book because I consider it to be a correct description of the material presented.

It is my hope that you will find this book to be beneficial to your knowledge and comprehension of basic EKG interpretation. Your suggestions and comments are welcome.

Brenda M. Beasley, RN, BS, EMT-Paramedic
Department Chair, Allied Health/EMS Program Director
Calhoun Community College
E-mail address: bjm18@aol.com

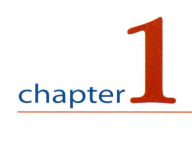

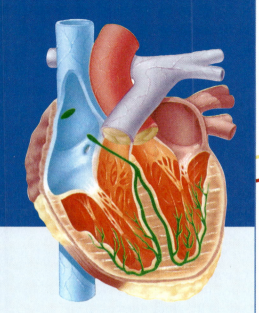

The Anatomy of the Heart: Structure

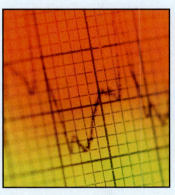

objectives

Upon completion of this chapter, the student will be able to:

➤ Describe the chambers of the heart
- a. Atria
- b. Ventricles

➤ Identify the location, shape, and size of the heart

➤ Name the layers of the heart

➤ Name the valves of the heart

➤ Describe the structure and function of the blood vessels
- a. Arteries
- b. Veins
- c. Capillaries

➤ Discuss the concept of pulmonary circulation

➤ Explain the concept of systemic circulation

INTRODUCTION

A thorough understanding of the structure of the heart provides the student with a foundation upon which to build the knowledge of basic dysrhythmia interpretation. Therefore, the focus of this chapter will be to provide you, the student, with a simple yet comprehensive look at cardiac anatomy. After you have mastered the knowledge of basic cardiac anatomy (structure), you will be prepared to move into Chapter 2, which addresses the basic physiology (function) of the heart.

ANATOMY OF THE HEART

First you must realize that the heart is a muscle. Although we don't think of exercising our heart muscle when we go to the gym, the fact is that your heart muscle (myocardium) is constantly in the "exercise mode." At times of rest, the exercise is more sedate. Think, however, of the vigor with which your heart muscle must exercise when you walk (or run) up six flights of stairs! Now as you feel your heart pumping, you can easily understand that your heart muscle is indeed exercising!

We often hear the heart referred to as a "two-sided pump," and this analogy works well in our understanding of the basics of cardiac anatomy. Indeed, one can visualize this pump as having a right side and a left side. On each side of the pump, there is an upper chamber of the heart, which is referred to as the **atrium (atria, plural)**, and a lower chamber of the heart known as the **ventricle**. In all, there are four hollow chambers in the normal heart. Again, the two upper chambers of the heart are called atria; the two lower chambers are called ventricles.

Separating the upper chambers is the interatrial septum. The lower, inferior chambers are separated by the interventricular septum. (See Figure 1–1.) Externally, the atrioventricular groove divides the atria from the ventricles. The anterior and posterior

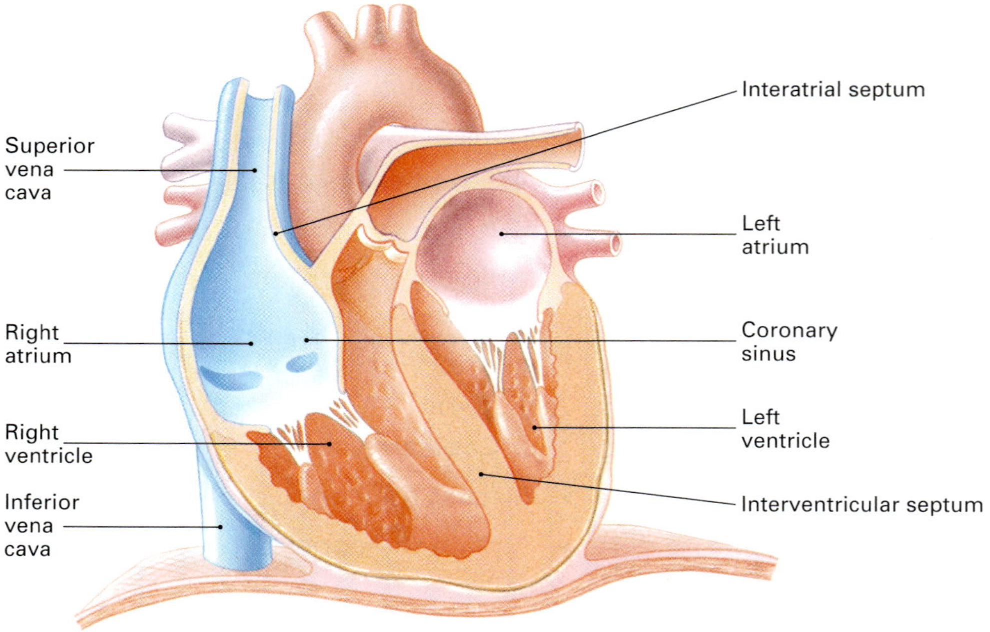

atrium upper chamber of the heart

ventricle lower chamber of the heart

Figure 1–1. The chambers of the heart

interventricular grooves separate the ventricles externally. The muscle fibers of the ventricles are continuous, as are the atrial muscle fibers.

The two upper chambers of the heart are located at the base, or top, of the heart; the lower chambers are located at the bottom, or apex, of the heart. The upper chambers of the heart are thin-walled and receive blood as it returns to the heart. The lower chambers of the heart have thicker walls and pump blood away from the heart, throughout the systemic circulation.

LOCATION, SIZE, AND SHAPE OF THE HEART

It is important for you to learn and understand the location of the heart in that the effectiveness of one of our most basic and most important skills—CPR—depends upon a reasonable knowledge of this position. In addition, the proper placement of electrodes to record an electrocardiogram, which will be discussed in Chapter 5, depends upon a proper understanding of the location of the heart.

The central section of the thorax (chest cavity) is called the **mediastinum**. It is in this area that the heart is housed, lying in front of the spinal column, behind the sternum, and between the lungs. (See Figure 1–2.)

mediastinum the central section of the thorax (chest cavity)

When thinking of the heart muscle in terms of its mass, one should realize that two-thirds of the heart muscle lies to the left of the midline. The apex of the heart lies just above the diaphragm. The base of the heart lies at approximately the level of the third rib. (Figures 1–2 and 1–4)

The exact size of the heart varies somewhat among individuals, but on average it is approximately 5 inches or 12 centimeters in length and 3 inches or 7.5 centimeters wide. The shape of the heart is somewhat conelike. It is appropriate to visualize the heart as approximately the size of the owner's closed fist. (See Figure 1–3.)

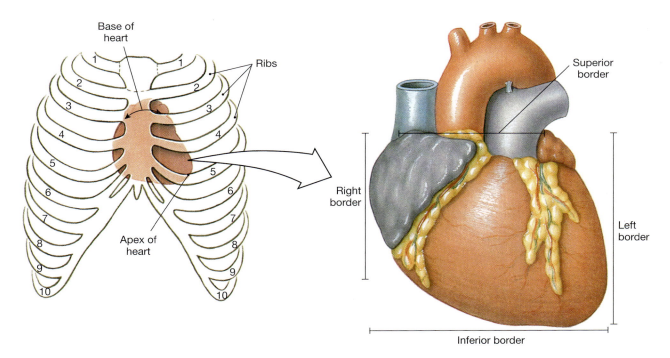

Figure 1–2. Position and orientation of the heart

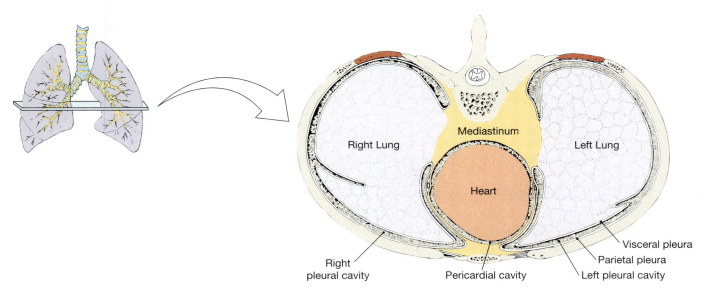

Figure 1–3. Anatomical relationships in the thoracic cavity

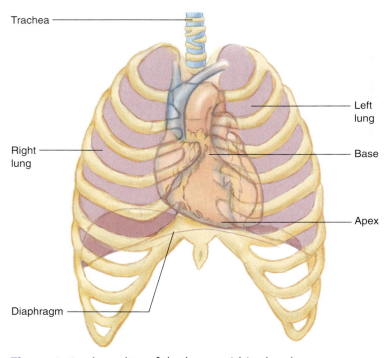

Figure 1–4. Location of the heart within the chest

LAYERS OF THE HEART

Pericardium

pericardium
closed, two-layered sac that surrounds the heart

Surrounding the heart is a closed, two-layered sac referred to as the **pericardium** or pericardial sac. In direct contact with the pleura is the outer layer or parietal pericardium. (See Figure 1–5.) This layer consists of tough, inelastic fibrous connective tissue and serves to prevent overdistention of the heart. The thin, serous inner layer of the peri-

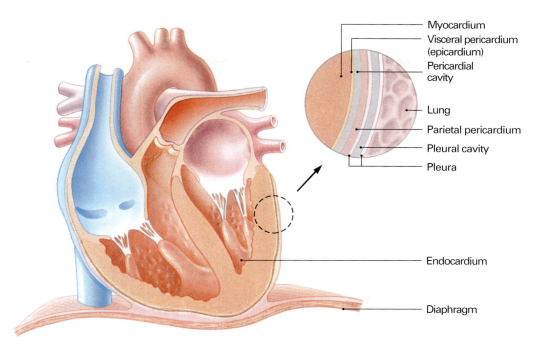

Myocardium
Visceral pericardium (epicardium)
Pericardial cavity
Lung
Parietal pericardium
Pleural cavity
Pleura
Endocardium
Diaphragm

Figure 1–5.   Layers of the heart

cardium is called the visceral pericardium and is contiguous with the epicardium, which surrounds the heart. The serous pericardium is considered a part of the heart and is continuous with the epicardium.

A space filled with a scant amount of fluid (approximately 10–20 cubic centimeters [cc]) separates the two pericardial layers. This fluid, by acting as a lubricant, helps to reduce friction as the heart moves within the pericardial sac.

An inflammation of the serous pericardium is called **pericarditis**. Although the cause of this disease is frequently unknown, it may result from infection or disease of the connective tissue. Pericarditis can cause severe pain, which may be confused with or mistaken for the pain of a myocardial infarction. This can make physical assessment of the patient a real challenge for the clinician.

Heart wall

Three primary layers of tissue compose the heart wall. This specialized cardiac muscle tissue is unique to the heart. The **epicardium** accounts for the smooth outer surface of the heart. The thick middle layer of the heart is called the **myocardium** and is the thickest of the three layers of the heart wall. The myocardium is composed primarily of cardiac muscle cells and is responsible for the heart's ability to contract. The innermost layer, the **endocardium,** is composed of thin connective tissue. This smooth inner surface of the heart and heart valves serves to allow blood to flow more easily throughout the heart.

VALVES OF THE HEART

The four valves of the heart allow blood to flow in only one direction. (See Figure 1–6.) There are two sets of valves, the atrioventricular valves and the semilunar valves.

pericarditis an inflammation of the serous pericardium

epicardium the smooth outer surface of the heart

myocardium the thick middle layer of the heart composed primarily of cardiac muscle cells and responsible for the heart's ability to contract

endocardium the innermost layer of the heart; composed of thin connective tissue

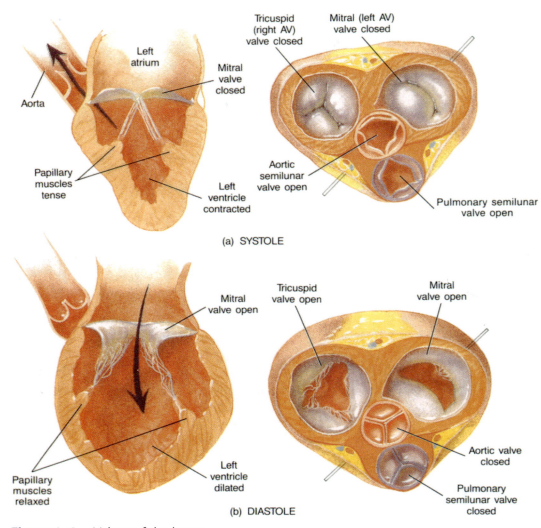

(a) SYSTOLE

(b) DIASTOLE

Figure 1–6. Valves of the heart

tricuspid valve named for its three cusps; located between the right atrium and the right ventricle

chordae tendineae fine chords of dense connective tissue that attach to papillary muscles in the wall of the ventricles

mitral (or bicuspid) valve similar in structure to the tricuspid valve but has only two cusps and is located between the left atrium and the left ventricle

Atrioventricular valves

As the term indicates, the atrioventricular valves are located between the atria and the ventricles. These valves allow blood to flow from the atria into the ventricles. They are also effective in preventing the blood from flowing backward from the ventricles into the atria. The **tricuspid valve** is named for its three cusps and is located between the right atrium and the right ventricle.

Free edges of each of the three cusps extend into the ventricles, where they attach to the chordae tendineae. **Chordae tendineae** are fine chords of dense connective tissue that attach to papillary muscles in the wall of the ventricles. Chordae tendineae and papillary muscles work in concert to prevent the cusps from fluttering back into the atrium and disrupting blood flow through the heart.

The **mitral (or bicuspid) valve** is similar in structure to the tricuspid valve but has only two cusps. The mitral valve is located between the left atrium and the left ventricle.

The mnemonic in Table 1–1 has proved helpful in recalling the location of the atrioventricular valves.

Table 1–1

Mnemonic: Heart valves	
Atrioventricular Valves	
L	Left
M	Mitral
R	Right
T	Tricuspid

Semilunar valves

Much as the atrioventricular valves prevent backflow of blood into the atria, the **semilunar valves** serve to prevent the backflow of blood into the ventricles. Each semilunar valve contains three semilunar (or moon-shaped) cusps. The semilunar valves are the pulmonic and aortic valves. The semilunar valve located between the right ventricle and the pulmonary artery is called the **pulmonic valve**. The semilunar valve located between the left ventricle and the trunk of the aorta is called the **aortic valve**.

Changes in chamber pressure govern the opening and closing of the heart valves. During ventricular systole (contraction of the ventricles), the atrioventricular valves close and the semilunar valves open. During ventricular diastole (relaxation of the ventricles), the aortic and pulmonic valves are closed and the mitral and tricuspid valves are open. Passive filling of the coronary arteries occurs during ventricular diastole.

ARTERIES, VEINS, AND CAPILLARIES

Since we tend to refer to the heart as the body's "pump," we can similarly consider the vasculature, or the blood vessels, as the "container" for the fluid, or blood. For the purposes of this text, it is appropriate to discuss three commonly accepted groups of blood vessels: arteries, veins, and capillaries.

Arteries

Arteries, by virtue of their primary function, are relatively thick-walled and muscular. These blood vessels function under high pressure in order to convey blood from the heart out to the rest of the body. The prefix "a" can mean "away from," and so it is helpful to remember that the word "artery" also begins with the letter "a"; thus arteries carry blood away from the heart. Larger arterial blood vessels are called arteries, and these vessels branch off into smaller blood vessels known as arterioles. Arteries carry oxygenated blood, with the exception of the pulmonary and umbilical arteries.

Arteries also operate in the regulation of blood pressure through functional changes in peripheral vascular resistance. Arterial walls consist of three distinct layers: the intima, media, and adventitia. (See Table 1–2 and Figure 1–7.) These layers are also

semilunar valves serve to prevent the backflow of blood into the ventricles and each valve contains three semilunar (or moon-shaped) cusps

pulmonic valve the semilunar valve located between the right ventricle and the pulmonary artery

aortic valve the semilunar valve located between the left ventricle and the trunk of the aorta

arteries thick-walled and muscular blood vessels that function under high pressure to convey blood from the heart out to the rest of the body

Table 1–2

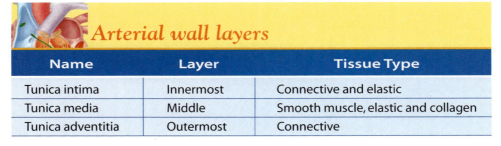

Name	Layer	Tissue Type
Tunica intima	Innermost	Connective and elastic
Tunica media	Middle	Smooth muscle, elastic and collagen
Tunica adventitia	Outermost	Connective

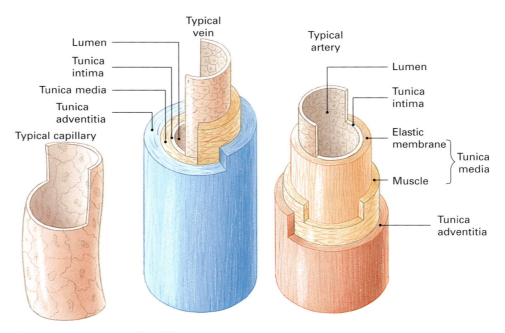

Figure 1–7. Arterial wall layers

called tunics (coats or coverings). The tunica intima is the innermost layer and consists of endothelium and an inner elastic membrane. This inner elastic membrane separates the intimal layer from the next layer, the tunica media. The tunica media is the middle layer and consists of smooth muscle cells. In this middle layer, the blood flow through the vessel is regulated by constriction or dilation. Vasoconstriction, a decrease in the diameter of the blood vessel, produces a decrease in blood flow. In contrast, vasodilation, an increase in the diameter of the blood vessel, produces an increase in blood flow. The tunica adventitia, or outermost layer, is composed of various connective tissues.

Other structures of importance for this discussion are the coronary arteries and the coronary sinus. The right and left coronary arteries arise from the trunk of the aorta and function to carry oxygenated blood throughout the myocardium. The coronary sinus (also referred to as the great cardiac vein) is a short trunk that serves to receive deoxygenated blood from the veins of the myocardium. This trunk empties into the right atrium. (See Figure 1–8.)

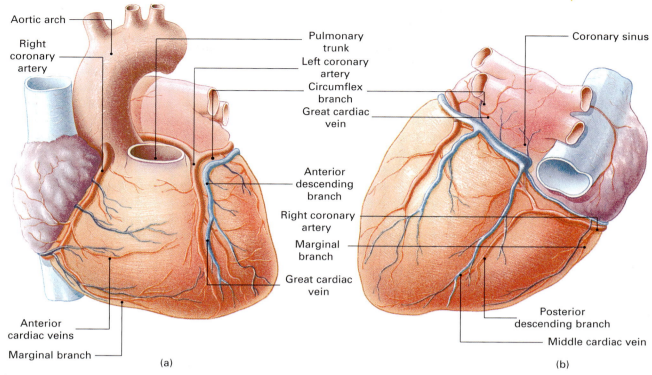

Right coronary artery

Figure 1–8.   Coronary circulation

Veins

Veins are defined as blood vessels that carry blood back to the heart. Veins branch off into smaller vessels known as venules. With the exception of venules, veins are structurally similar to arteries in that they also have three layers. Unlike arteries, however, veins operate under low pressure, are relatively thin-walled, and contain one-way valves. With the exception of the pulmonary vein, the veins convey deoxygenated blood.

The larger veins of the body ultimately empty into the two largest veins, the **superior vena cava** and the **inferior vena cava**, which empty deoxygenated blood into the heart's right atrium. The superior vena cava drains blood from the head and neck. The inferior vena cava collects blood from the rest of the body (See Figure 1–9.)

Capillaries

Capillaries are tiny blood vessels whose walls are the thinnest of all blood vessels. There is a greater number of capillaries in the human body than of any other blood vessel. In fact, capillaries are so tiny that red blood cells must "march through" in single file. From the arterioles, blood flows into the capillaries, where the vast majority of gas exchange occurs.

In summary, arterioles transport oxygenated blood into the capillaries. Capillaries allow for the exchange of oxygen, nutrients, and waste products between the blood and body tissues and are viewed as "connectors" between arteries and veins. The smallest of the veins, the venules, then receive the deoxygenated blood, which travels back to the heart via the venous system. To get a clearer picture of blood flow through the various vessels, please refer to Figure 1–10.

veins blood vessels that carry blood back to the heart, operate under low pressure, and are relatively thin-walled

superior vena cava drains blood from the head and neck

inferior vena cava collects blood from the rest of the body

capillaries tiny blood vessels that allow for the exchange of oxygen, nutrients, and waste products between the blood and body tissues; "connectors" between arteries and veins

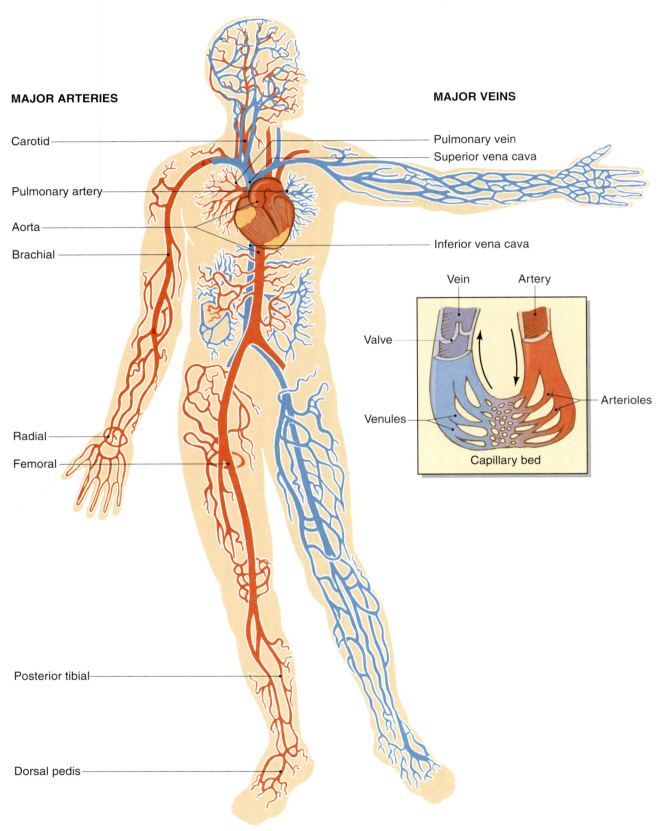

MAJOR ARTERIES

Carotid

Pulmonary artery

Aorta

Brachial

Radial

Femoral

Posterior tibial

Dorsal pedis

MAJOR VEINS

Pulmonary vein

Superior vena cava

Inferior vena cava

Vein

Artery

Valve

Venules

Arterioles

Capillary bed

Figure 1–9. Circulatory system

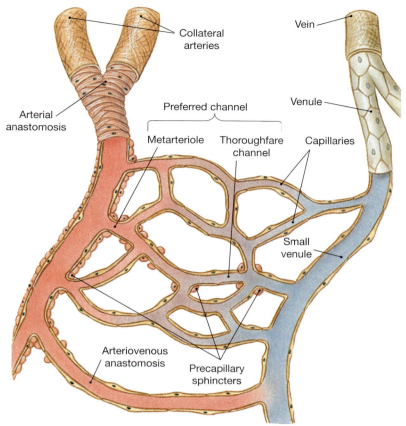

Figure 1–10.   Organization of capillary bed

This chapter would not be complete without a brief discussion of the circulatory system. **Circulation** refers to movement through a course (the body) which leads back to the initial point (the heart). Two major components compose the circulatory system, the pulmonary circulation and the systemic circulation.

PULMONARY CIRCULATION

A rudimentary way to remember pulmonary circulation is to recall that it is the blood flow between the heart and lungs. When blood leaves the heart through the right ventricle and travels into the pulmonary artery to the lungs and back through the pulmonary veins to the left atrium, the cycle is known as **pulmonary circulation**. The importance of this component of the circulatory system cannot be overemphasized. The critical concept of tissue perfusion is based on adequate gas exchange within the alveolar capillary membranes in the lungs.

SYSTEMIC CIRCULATION

Systemic circulation consists of the circulation of blood as it leaves the left ventricle and travels through the arteries, capillaries, and veins of the entire body system and back to the primary receptacle of the heart (the right atrium). Maintenance of each

circulation
movement through a course (the body) which leads back to the initial point (the heart)

pulmonary circulation when blood leaves the heart through the right ventricle and travels into the pulmonary artery to the lungs and back through the pulmonary veins to the left atrium

systemic circulation the circulation of blood as it leaves the left ventricle and travels through the arteries, capillaries, and veins of the entire body system and back to the primary receptacle of the heart (the right atrium)

tissue type in the body is ensured by the work of the systemic and pulmonary circulations, collectively.

SUMMARY

Your understanding of the anatomy of the heart and blood vessels will become increasingly important as you move from chapter to chapter in this book. It is not possible to have a thorough understanding of dysrhythmias and their causes unless you also have a good grasp of cardiovascular anatomy.

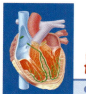

Review Questions
CHAPTER 1

1. The fibrous sac covering of the heart, which is in contact with the pleura, is the:
   a. Epicardium
   b. Myocardium
   c. Pericardium
   d. Endocardium

2. The lower chamber of the heart, with the thickest myocardium, is the:
   a. Right
   b. Left

3. The pulmonic and aortic valves are open during:
   a. Systole
   b. Diastole

4. The large blood vessel that returns unoxygenated blood from the head and neck to the right atrium is called the:
   a. Jugular vein
   b. Carotid artery
   c. Superior vena cava
   d. Inferior vena cava

5. The innermost layer of the arterial wall is called the:
   a. Tunica intima
   b. Tunica media
   c. Myocardium
   d. Tunica adventitia

6. The most numerous blood vessels in the body are the:
   a. Arteries
   b. Capillaries
   c. Venules
   d. Veins

7. Blood flow between the heart and lungs is _____ circulation.
   a. Systemic
   b. Venous
   c. Myocardial
   d. Pulmonary

8. These blood vessels function under high pressure in order to convey blood from the heart out to the rest of the body:
   a. Venules
   b. Veins
   c. Arteries
   d. Capillaries

9. An inflammation of the serous pericardium is called:
   a. Myocarditis
   b. Pericarditis
   c. Pulmonitis
   d. Tendonitis

10. The smooth outer surface of the heart is called the:
    a. Pericardium
    b. Endocardium
    c. Epicardium
    d. Myocardium

11. The _____ valve is named for its three cusps and is located between the right atrium and the right ventricle.
    a. Bicuspid
    b. Tricuspid
    c. Aortic
    d. Pulmonic

12. Chordae tendineae and papillary muscles work in concert to prevent the cusps from fluttering back into the:
    a. Atrium
    b. Ventricle
    c. Aorta
    d. Vena cava

13. The right and left coronary arteries arise from the:
    a. Left ventricle
    b. Right atrium
    c. Coronary sinus
    d. Trunk of the aorta

14. The central section of the thorax (chest cavity) is called the:
    a. Costal margin
    b. Mediastinum
    c. Diaphragm
    d. Xiphoid

15. The apex of the heart lies just above the:

    a. Intercostal space

    b. Mediastinum

    c. Diaphragm

    d. Xiphoid

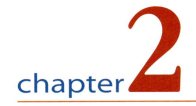

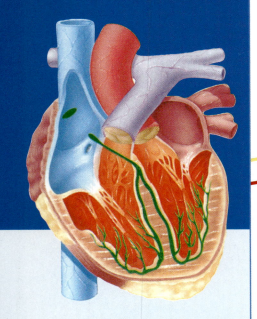

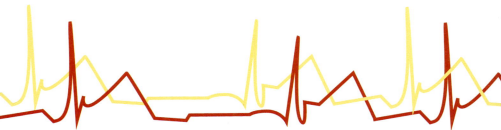

Cardiovascular Physiology: Function

objectives

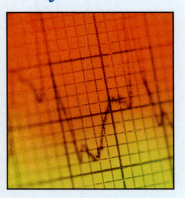

Upon completion of this chapter, the student will be able to:

➤ Describe the sequence of blood flow through the heart

➤ Describe the cardiac cycle, including

   a. Definition

   b. Systole

   c. Diastole

➤ Discuss the term "stroke volume"

➤ Discuss cardiac output, preload, Starling's law, and afterload

➤ Describe the autonomic nervous system

INTRODUCTION

Now that we have addressed the structure of the heart, we will discuss the basic function, or physiology, of the cardiovascular system. We will build on the foundation provided in Chapters 1 and 2 as we sequentially discuss each chapter in order to gain a thorough knowledge of interpreting basic dysrhythmias. The focus of this chapter will be to provide you, the student, with an uncomplicated yet inclusive look at cardiac physiology. After you have mastered the knowledge of basic cardiac physiology, or function, you will be prepared to move on to Chapter 3, which addresses the basic electrophysiology of the heart.

NOTE: Now is the perfect time to look back at the review questions from Chapter 1. Then proceed on through the objectives and contents of this chapter.

BLOOD FLOW THROUGH THE HEART

The path of blood flow through the heart (Figure 2–1.) is our first consideration in acquiring knowledge of the physiology of circulation. Imagine, if you will, that the right atrium is a receptacle functioning in part to receive unoxygenated blood from the head,

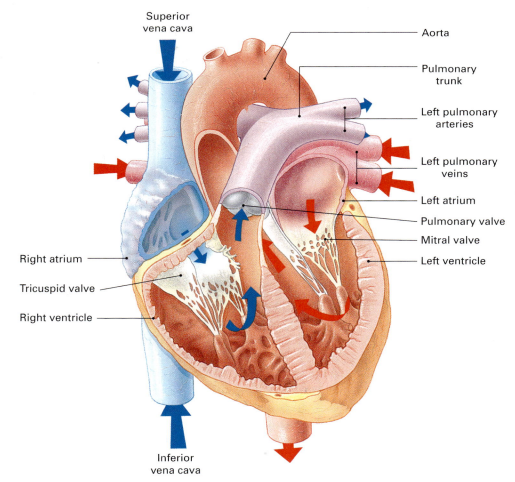

Figure 2–1. Blood flow through the heart

neck, and trunk. In order to simplify the route of circulation, the learner may choose to divide this concept into three components.

The first component would consist of blood flow through the right atrium, which proceeds as follows. Unoxygenated blood flows from the inferior and superior vena cava into the:

Right atrium	Through the tricuspid valve	Into the right ventricle	Through the pulmonic valve

The second component of blood flow through the pulmonary circulation continues when the blood travels from the pulmonic valve into the:

Pulmonary arteries	Into the lungs	Through the pulmonary alveolar-capillary network	Into the pulmonary veins

The third and final component of blood flow through the pulmonary circulation continues when the blood travels from the pulmonary veins into the:

Left atrium	Through the mitral valve	Into the left ventricle	Through the aortic valve and out to the rest of the body

It should be noted that the freshly oxygenated blood, traveling through the aortic valve, also enters the coronary arteries during diastole, when the aortic valve closes, to accomplish myocardial oxygenation. The vital function of gas exchange occurs in the second or middle component of pulmonary circulation when carbon dioxide is exchanged for oxygen in the pulmonary alveolar-capillary network.

CARDIAC CYCLE

cardiac cycle the actual time sequence between ventricular contraction and ventricular relaxation

systole, or **ventricular systole,** is consistent with the simultaneous contraction of the ventricles

diastole is synonymous with ventricular relaxation

The heart functions as a unit in that both atria contract simultaneously, then both ventricles contract. (See Figure 2–2.) When the atria contract, the ventricles are filled to their limit. Blood is ejected into the pulmonary and systemic circulations when simultaneous contraction of the ventricles occurs. At the time of ventricular contraction, the mitral and tricuspid valves are closed by the pressure of the contraction, while the pulmonic and aortic valves are opened. The **cardiac cycle** represents the actual time sequence between ventricular contraction and ventricular relaxation.

Systole, also referred to as **ventricular systole,** is consistent with the simultaneous contraction of the ventricles, while **diastole** is synonymous with ventricular relaxation. The ventricles fill passively with approximately 70 percent of the blood that has collected in the atria during ventricular diastole. Then the active contraction of the atria propels the remaining 30 percent of the blood into the ventricles. Atrial contraction has only a minimal role in filling; consequently, even if the atria do not contract effectively,

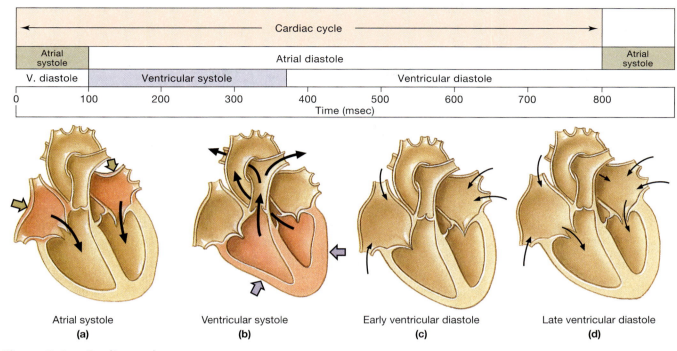

Figure 2–2.   Cardiac cycle

ventricular filling still ensues. During periods of ventricular relaxation, cardiac filling and coronary perfusion occur passively.

One cardiac cycle occurs every 0.8 second. Systole lasts about 0.28 second. Diastole lasts about 0.52 second. Therefore, the period of diastole is substantially longer than the period of systole.

STROKE VOLUME

Stroke volume may be defined as the volume of blood pumped out of one ventricle of the heart in a single beat or contraction. Stroke volume is estimated at approximately 70 cc (cubic centimeters, or milliliters) per beat. The number of contractions, or beats, per minute of the heart is known as the **heart rate.** The normal adult heart rate is 60–100 beats per minute.

CARDIAC OUTPUT

Cardiac output is the amount of blood pumped by the left ventricle in 1 minute. Ventricle outputs are considered to be normally equal, because these two chambers contract simultaneously.

By remembering the following formula, we can determine the cardiac output:

stroke volume
the volume of blood pumped out of one ventricle of the heart in a single beat or contraction

heart rate the number of contractions, or beats, per minute of the heart

cardiac output
the amount of blood pumped by the left ventricle in 1 minute

| Cardiac output (CO) = | Stroke volume (SV) × heart rate (HR) |

Consequently, if a patient has a heart rate of 80 beats per minute (bpm) and a stroke volume of 70 cc per beat, the resulting cardiac output will be approximately 5600 cc per minute (or 5.6 liters per minute). When, for any of a variety of reasons, a patient's cardiac output is outside the normal range, the heart will try to balance it by changes in either the stroke volume or the heart rate.

Inadequate cardiac output may be indicated by any combination of the following signs and symptoms: shortness of breath, dizziness, decreased blood pressure, chest pains, and cool and clammy skin. Note that patients may exhibit other signs and symptoms as well. If your patient complains of chest pain and begins to exhibit any of the signs and symptoms of inadequate cardiac output, you should immediately contact a physician.

Commonly called end-diastolic pressure, **preload** is the pressure in the ventricles at the end of diastole. **Afterload** is the resistance against which the heart must pump. This pressure also affects stroke volume and cardiac output.

When the volume of blood in the ventricles is increased, this causes stretching of the ventricular myocardial fibers and consequently a more forceful contraction. This concept is known as **Starling's law of the heart.** This concept is a law of physiology: that basically, the more the myocardial fibers are stretched, up to a certain point, the more forceful the subsequent contraction will be. Thus we can assume that if the volume of blood filling the ventricle increases significantly, so will the force of the cardiac contraction. This may be thought of as analogous to the stretching of a rubber band; thus we have the "rubber band theory": the farther you stretch a rubber band, the harder it snaps back to its original size.

The amount of opposition to blood flow offered by the arterioles is known as **peripheral vascular resistance (PVR)** or systemic vascular resistance (SVR). A patient's blood pressure may increase or decrease if the cardiac output changes significantly and the peripheral vascular resistance remains uniform. Vasoconstriction and vasodilation determine peripheral vascular resistance. Blood pressure is subject to change if the cardiac output or peripheral vascular resistance changes.

Therefore, it may be helpful to remember the following formula:

Blood pressure (BP) =	Cardiac output (CO) × peripheral vascular resistance (PVR)

AUTONOMIC NERVOUS SYSTEM

When we consider all the pathophysiological processes that are required in order to maintain homeostasis, or equilibrium, in the internal environment of our bodies, we quickly realize that we are fortunate to possess a built-in control center. This control center is known as the **autonomic nervous system.**

The autonomic nervous system regulates functions of the body that are involuntary, or not under conscious control. In other words, we do not have to consciously think about our every heartbeat or about regulating our blood pressure. Heart rate and blood pressure are regulated by this component of the nervous system. (See Figure 2–3.)

There are two major divisions of the autonomic nervous system: the sympathetic nervous system and the parasympathetic nervous system. The majority of organs in the body are innervated by both systems. It is important to note that blood vessels are innervated only by the sympathetic nervous system. The **sympathetic nervous system** is responsible for preparation of the body for physical activity ("fight or flight"). The

preload the pressure in the ventricles at the end of diastole

afterload the resistance against which the heart must pump

Starling's law of the heart the more the myocardial fibers are stretched, up to a certain point, the more forceful the subsequent contraction will be

peripheral vascular resistance (PVR) the amount of opposition to blood flow offered by the arterioles

autonomic nervous system regulates functions of the body that are involuntary, or not under conscious control

sympathetic nervous system responsible for preparation of the body for physical activity ("fight or flight")

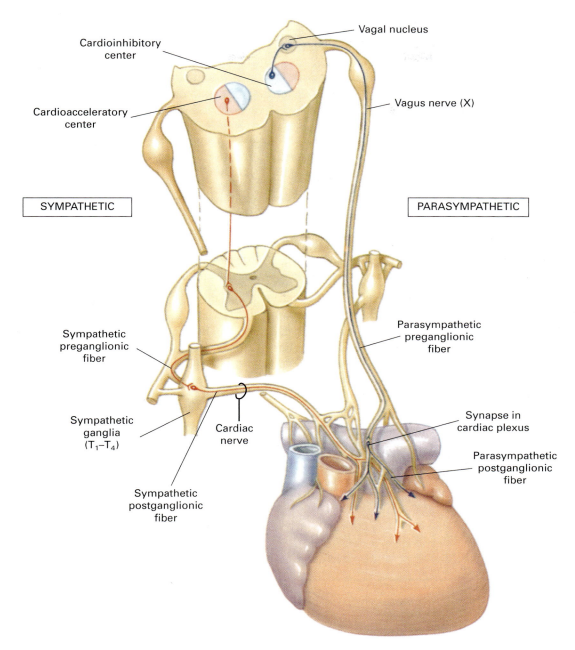

Figure 2–3. Nervous control of the heart

parasympathetic nervous system regulates the calmer functions ("rest and digest") of our existence.

RECEPTORS AND NEUROTRANSMITTERS

Nerve endings of the sympathetic nervous system and the parasympathetic nervous system secrete neurotransmitters. The sympathetic nervous system has two types of receptor fibers at the nerve endings. The receptors are the alpha- and beta-receptors. The

parasympathetic nervous system regulates the calmer ("rest and digest") functions

norepinephrine
the chemical neurotransmitter for the sympathetic nervous system

acetylcholine
the chemical neurotransmitter for the parasympathetic nervous system

chemical neurotransmitter for the sympathetic nervous system is **norepinephrine**. These nerve endings are called adrenergic. When norepinephrine is released, an increase in heart rate and contractile force of cardiac fibers and vasoconstriction will result.

The chemical neurotransmitter for the parasympathetic nervous system is **acetylcholine,** and the nerve endings are known as cholinergic. When acetylcholine is released, the heart rate slows, as does the atrioventricular conduction rate. With the exception of capillaries, all the body's blood vessels have alpha-adrenergic receptors, whereas the heart and lungs have beta-adrenergic receptors.

Understanding adrenergic receptors and their effects on heart rate

For the sake of simplicity, we will discuss only the basics of the receptors and neuro-transmitters. Let's first consider some rudimentary definitions:

Adrenergic—of or pertaining to the sympathetic nerve fibers of the autonomic nervous system that use epinephrine or epinephrine-like (norepinephrine) substances as neurotransmitters.

Receptor—reactive site on the cell surface or within the cell that combines with a drug molecule to produce a physiological effect.

Cholinergic—of or pertaining to the parasympathetic nerve fibers of the autonomic nervous system that use acetylcholine as the neurotransmitter.

The effects of the alpha- and beta-receptors can be briefly described as follows (see also Table 2–1):

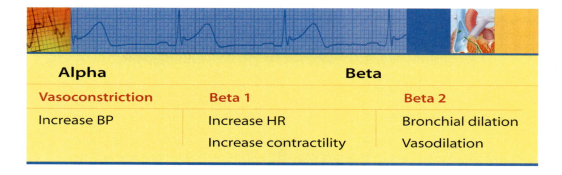

Alpha	Beta	
Vasoconstriction	**Beta 1**	**Beta 2**
Increase BP	Increase HR	Bronchial dilation
	Increase contractility	Vasodilation

Remember A B C D!

A B C D = *Alpha* Constricts, *Beta* Dilates

Table 2–1

Organs affected by alpha- and beta-receptors:

Organs affected	Alpha	Beta 1	Beta 2
Heart	Yes	Yes	No
Lungs	No	No	Yes
Vessels	Yes	No	Yes

SUMMARY

It is important to understand not only the structure of the cardiovascular system, but also the function of the various structures. Indeed, it would be difficult to understand just why a particular component of the heart had ceased to function properly unless you were familiar with the proper or "normal" function of that component. Thus, this chapter has focused on simplifying a very complicated subject, cardiovascular physiology.

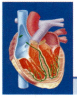

Review Questions

CHAPTER 2

1. The left side of the heart is a low-pressure pump.

   a. True

   b. False

2. The major blood vessel that receives blood from the head and upper extremities and transports it to the heart is the:

   a. Trunk of the aorta

   b. Superior vena cava

   c. Inferior vena cava

   d. Pulmonary artery

3. The course of blood flow through the heart and lungs is referred to as _____ circulation.

   a. Aortic

   b. Pulmonary

   c. Systemic

   d. Collateral

4. Cardiac output is a factor of which of the elements below?

   a. Cardiac rate

   b. Stroke volume

   c. Partial vascular resistance

   d. A and b

5. The chief chemical neurotransmitter for the parasympathetic nervous system is:

   a. Acetylcholine

   b. Norepinephrine

   c. Epinephrine

   d. Atropine

6. The heart has _____ chambers.

   a. Two

   b. Three

   c. Four

   d. Six

7. The chief chemical neurotransmitter for the sympathetic nervous system is:

   a. Acetylcholine

   b. Norepinephrine

c. Ephedrine

d. Atropine

8. Unoxygenated blood flows from the inferior and superior vena cavae into the:

   a. Left atrium

   b. Left ventricle

   c. Right ventricle

   d. Right atrium

9. One cardiac cycle occurs every:

   a. 0.8 second

   b. 0.5 second

   c. 0.52 second

   d. 1.2 seconds

10. With the exception of _____, all the body's blood vessels have alpha-adrenergic receptors whereas the heart and lungs have beta-adrenergic receptors.

   a. Arterioles

   b. Capillaries

   c. Venules

   d. Aorta

11. Blood travels from the left atrium through the _____ valve and into the left ventricle.

   a. Aortic

   b. Pulmonic

   c. Bicuspid

   d. Tricuspid

12. Blood travels from the right atrium through the _____ valve and into the right ventricle.

   a. Aortic

   b. Pulmonic

   c. Bicuspid

   d. Tricuspid

13. Starling's law of the heart is also referred to as:

   a. Cushing's theory

   b. Beck's triad

   c. The rubber band theory

   d. The Hering-Breuer reflex

INTRODUCTION

Although an in-depth study of cardiac electrophysiology can be quite complicated and baffling to the novice student, the intent of this text is to concentrate on the **basics** of interpreting dysrhythmias. Thus this discussion of electrophysiology will center on rudimentary, but very important, concepts.

In our discussion of cardiac anatomy in Chapter 1, we established that the heart is a unique and distinctive organ, unlike any other in the human body. The heart is composed of cardiac muscle, which is made up of thousands of myocardial cells. For the purposes of our discussion, we will note that there are two basic myocardial cell groups: the myocardial working cells and the specialized pacemaker cells of the electrical conduction system.

BASIC CELL GROUPS

Myocardial working cells

myocardial working cells responsible for generating the physical contraction of the heart muscle

The **myocardial working cells** are responsible for generating the physical contraction of the heart muscle. The muscular layer of the wall of the atria and the thicker muscular layer of the ventricular walls are constructed of myocardial working cells. Myocardial working cells are permeated by contractile filaments, which, when electrically stimulated, produce myocardial contraction. Thus the primary functions of the myocardial working cells include both contraction and relaxation.

It should be noted that this physical contraction of myocardial tissue actually generates blood flow; however, organized electrical activity is required in order to produce the physical contraction. As the myocardial tissue contracts, the size of the atria and ventricles decreases, so that blood is ejected from the chambers.

Specialized pacemaker cells

specialized group responsible for controlling the rate and rhythm of the heart by coordinating regular depolarization and are found in the electrical conduction system of the heart

threshold refers to the point at which a stimulus will produce a cell response

Unlike the myocardial working cells, the specialized pacemaker cells of the electrical conduction system do not contain contractile filaments and thus do not have the ability to contract. Rather, the cells in this **specialized group** are responsible for controlling the rate and rhythm of the heart by coordinating regular depolarization. These cells are found in the electrical conduction system of the heart. Thus the generation and the conduction of electrical impulses are the primary functions of the specialized myocardial pacemaker cells.

Cardiac muscle cells have the ability to contract in response to thermal, chemical, electrical, or mechanical stimuli. All atrial muscle cells contract simultaneously; comparably, all ventricular muscle cells contract together.

The term **threshold** refers to the point at which a stimulus will produce a cell response. When a stimulus is strong enough for cardiac cells to reach the threshold, all cells will respond to this stimulus and will thus contract. This action is known as the "all-or-none" phenomenon of cardiac muscle cells; that is, all cells will respond or none will respond. Hence, cardiac muscle functions on an all-or-none principle.

PRIMARY CARDIAC CELL CHARACTERISTICS

Cardiac cells have four primary cell characteristics. (See Table 3–1.) These properties are excitability (or irritability), conductivity, contractility (or rhythmicity), and automaticity. Only one of these characteristics, contractility, is considered a mechanical

Table 3–1

Primary cardiac cell characteristics

Characteristic	Location	Function
Automaticity	SA node, AV junction, Purkinje network fibers	Electrical
Excitability	All cardiac cells	Electrical
Conductivity	All cardiac cells	Electrical
Contractility	Myocardial muscle cells	Mechanical

function of the heart. The other three characteristics—automaticity, excitability, and conductivity—are electrical functions of the heart.

Automaticity is the ability of cardiac pacemaker cells to generate their own electrical impulses spontaneously without external (or nervous) stimulation. This intrinsic spontaneous depolarization frequency produces contraction of myocardial muscle cells. This characteristic is specific to the pacemaker cell sites of the electrical conduction system (i.e., the SA node, the AV junction, and the Purkinje network fibers).

Excitability—or irritability—is the ability of cardiac cells to respond to an electrical stimulus. This characteristic is shared by all cardiac cells. A weaker stimulus can cause a contraction when a cardiac cell is highly irritable.

Conductivity is the ability of cardiac cells to receive an electrical stimulus and then transmit it other cardiac cells. This characteristic is shared by all cardiac cells because these cells are connected together to form a syncytium; that is, they function collectively as a unit. In referring to more than one of these units, the correct term is "syncytia."

Contractility, also referred to as rhythmicity, is the ability of cardiac cells to shorten and cause cardiac muscle contraction in response to an electrical stimulus. Contractility can be thought of as the coordination of contractions of cardiac muscle cells to produce a regular heartbeat. Through the administration of certain medications, such as dopamine and epinephrine, cardiac contractility can be strengthened.

MAJOR ELECTROLYTES THAT AFFECT CARDIAC FUNCTION

Because myocardial cells are bathed in electrolyte solutions, both mechanical and electrical cardiac function are influenced by electrolyte imbalances. An **electrolyte** is a substance or compound whose molecules dissociate into charged components, or ions, when placed in water, producing positively and negatively charged ions. An ion with a positive charge is called a **cation**, and an ion with a negative charge is called an **anion**.

The three major cations that affect cardiac function are potassium (K), sodium (Na), and calcium (Ca). Magnesium (Mg) is also an important cation. Potassium, magnesium, and calcium are intracellular (inside the cell) cations whereas sodium is an extracellular (outside the cell) cation.

Potassium performs a major function in cardiac depolarization and repolarization. An increase in potassium blood levels is known as hyperkalemia; a potassium deficit is hypokalemia.

Sodium plays a vital part in depolarization of the myocardium. An increase in sodium blood levels is known as hypernatremia; a sodium deficit is hyponatremia.

automaticity the ability of cardiac pacemaker cells to generate their own electrical impulses spontaneously without external (or nervous) stimulation

excitability the ability of cardiac cells to respond to an electrical stimulus, a characteristic shared by all cardiac cells

conductivity the ability of cardiac cells to receive an electrical stimulus and then transmit it to other cardiac cells

contractility, also referred to as rhythmicity, is the ability of cardiac cells to shorten and cause cardiac muscle contraction in response to an electrical stimulus

electrolyte a substance or compound whose molecules dissociate into charged components, or ions, when placed in water, producing positively and negatively charged ions

cation an ion with a positive charge

anion an ion with a negative charge

Calcium has an important function in myocardial depolarization and myocardial contraction. An increase in calcium blood levels is known as hypercalcemia; a calcium deficit is defined as hypocalcemia.

MOVEMENT OF IONS

Let's think now about the cardiac cells at rest, or in their resting state. Normally there is an ionic difference on the two sides of the cell membrane. In this state, potassium ion concentration is greater inside the cell than outside, and sodium ion concentration is greater outside the cell than inside. Potassium ions can diffuse through the membrane more readily than can sodium ions. By means of an active, or energized, mechanism of transport called the **sodium-potassium exchange pump,** potassium and sodium ions are moved in and out of the cell through the cell membrane. During the polarized, or resting, state, the inside of the cell is electrically negative relative to the outside of the cell. For the purposes of our discussions in the upcoming chapters, it should be noted that during this resting period a baseline or isoelectric line is recorded on the EKG strip.

CARDIAC DEPOLARIZATION

When an impulse develops and spreads throughout the myocardium, certain changes occur in the heart muscle fibers. These changes are referred to as cardiac depolarization and cardiac repolarization. In order to interpret an EKG accurately and reasonably, one must understand the concept of cardiac depolarization and repolarization.

First we will define a few terms which will be used in this discussion.

Resting membrane potential—state of a cardiac cell in which the inside of the cell membrane is negative compared with the outside of the cell membrane; exists when cardiac cells are in the resting state.

Action potential—change in polarity; a five-phase cycle that produces changes in the cell membrane's electrical charge; caused by stimulation of myocardial cells which extends across the myocardium; propagated in an all-or-none fashion.

Syncytium—cardiac muscle cell groups that are connected together and function collectively as a unit.

Polarized state—resting state of a cardiac cell, wherein the inside of the cell is electrically negative relative to the outside of the cell.

Depolarization—electrical occurrence normally expected to result in myocardial contraction; involves the movement of ions across cardiac cell membranes, resulting in positive polarity inside the cell membrane.

Repolarization—process whereby the depolarized cell is polarized and positive charges are again on the outside and negative charges on the inside of the cell; a return to the resting state.

For clarity, cardiac depolarization may be thought of as the period during which sodium ions rush into the cell, changing the interior charge to positive, after a myocardial cell has been stimulated. Recall now that this change of polarity is referred to as the **action potential.** In an effort to change the interior cell polarity to positive, calcium also slowly enters the cell. This activated state of the myocardial cells now spreads through the syncytium, followed closely by myocardial muscle contraction. This difference in the electric charge, or polarity, on the outside of the cell membrane results in the flow of electric current, which is recorded as waveforms on the EKG. (See Figure 3–1.)

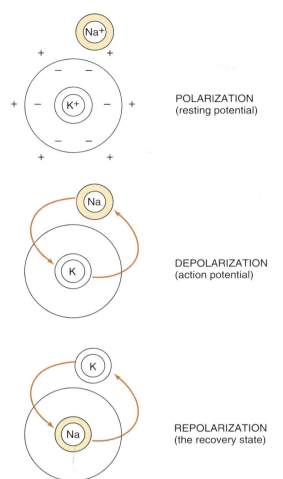

POLARIZATION
(resting potential)

DEPOLARIZATION
(action potential)

REPOLARIZATION
(the recovery state)

Figure 3–1.   Ion shifts during depolarization and repolarization

CARDIAC REPOLARIZATION

At the end of cardiac depolarization, the sodium actively returns to the outside of the cell, and potassium returns to the inside of the cell. This exchange takes place via the sodium-potassium exchange pump. The cell has now returned to the recovered, or re-polarized, state. The cardiac cell is now ready to be stimulated again. Repolarization is a slower process than depolarization.

It may be helpful to recall that the polarized cell is in the resting state, the depo-larized cell is utilizing its action potential, and the repolarized cell is in the recovery phase. It should be noted that the last area to be depolarized is the first area to be repo-larized in normal, healthy cardiac muscle.

REFRACTORY PERIODS

Like all other excitable tissue, cardiac muscle tissue has a refractory period to ensure that the muscle is totally relaxed before another action potential or depolarization can be initiated. The refractory period of atrial muscle (approximately 0.15 second) is much shorter than that of the ventricular muscle (approximately 0.25–0.3 second). Thus the rate of atrial contractions can potentially be much faster than that of the ventricles.

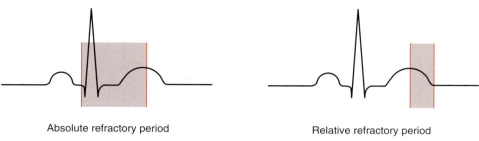

Absolute refractory period   Relative refractory period

Figure 3–2. Refractory periods

After electrical impulse stimulation and myocardial contraction, the cardiac cells have a brief resting period. As we learned earlier in this discussion, this period of rest is referred to as cardiac repolarization. During this state of repolarization, the heart goes through two stages: the absolute refractory period and the relative refractory period. (See Figure 3–2.)

During most of the process of repolarization, the cardiac cell is unable to respond to a new electrical stimulus. In addition, the cardiac cell cannot spontaneously depolarize. This stage of cell activity is referred to as the **absolute refractory period**. Remember that, regardless of the strength of the stimulus, the cardiac cell cannot be stimulated to depolarize in this period. The absolute refractory period corresponds with the beginning of the QRS complex to the peak of the T wave on the EKG strip.

The second part of the refractory period follows the absolute refractory period and is referred to as the **relative refractory period**. This is the period when repolarization is almost complete, and the cardiac cell can be stimulated to contract prematurely if the stimulus is much stronger than normal. On the EKG strip, the relative refractory period corresponds with the downslope of the T wave. The relative refractory period is also known as the vulnerable period of the cardiac cells during repolarization.

SUMMARY

As you began to comprehend, through your study of Chapters 1 and 2, the heart is a unique organ, unlike any other in the human body. You should now understand that the heart is composed of cardiac muscle made up of thousands of myocardial cells. In this chapter, we discussed the two basic myocardial cell groups: the myocardial working cells and the specialized pacemaker cells of the electrical conduction system.

absolute refractory period stage of cell activity in which the cardiac cell cannot spontaneously depolarize

relative refractory period the period when repolarization is almost complete, and the cardiac cell can be stimulated to contract prematurely if the stimulus is much stronger than normal

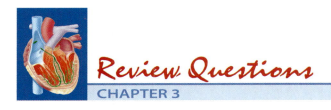

Review Questions

CHAPTER 3

1. The primary functions of the myocardial working cells include:
   a. Automaticity
   b. Regeneration
   c. Contraction and relaxation
   d. Impulse propagation

2. The ability of cardiac pacemaker cells to generate their own electrical impulses spontaneously without external, or nervous, stimulation is known as:
   a. Automaticity
   b. Contractility
   c. Conductility
   d. Action potential

3. Which characteristic is specific to the pacemaker sites of the electrical conduction system (i.e., the SA node, the AV junction, and the Purkinje network fibers)?
   a. Automaticity
   b. Contractility
   c. Conductility
   d. Excitability

4. The ability of cardiac cells to respond to an electrical stimulus is referred to as:
   a. Automaticity
   b. Contractility
   c. Conductility
   d. Excitability

5. Excitability is also referred to as:
   a. Irritability
   b. Automaticity
   c. Contractility
   d. Conductility

6. The ability of cardiac cells to receive an electrical stimulus and then transmit the stimulus to other cardiac cells is known as:
   a. Irritability
   b. Automaticity
   c. Contractility
   d. Conductivity

7. Conductivity is a characteristic shared by all cardiac cells.

   a. True

   b. False

8. Cardiac muscle cell groups that function collectively as a unit are known as:

   a. Syncytia

   b. Refractory

   c. Electrical

   d. Bundles

9. Repolarization is a slower process than depolarization.

   a. True

   b. False

10. The period when repolarization is almost complete and the cardiac cell can be stimulated to contract prematurely if the stimulus is stronger than normal is known as:

    a. The relative refractory period

    b. The absolute refractory period

    c. The action potential phase

    d. Absolute depolarization

11. Cardiac depolarization may be thought of as the period during which _____ ions rush into the cell.

    a. Potassium

    b. Calcium

    c. Sodium

    d. Chloride

12. At the end of cardiac depolarization, _____ ions return to the inside of the cell.

    a. Potassium

    b. Calcium

    c. Sodium

    d. Magnesium

13. The resting state of a cardiac cell, wherein the inside of the cell is electrically negative relative to the outside of the cell, is called:

    a. Active state

    b. Polarized state

    c. Depolarization

    d. Repolarization

14.   The point at which a stimulus will produce a cell response is called the:

   a.   Active state

   b.   All-or-none phase

   c.   Threshold

   d.   Rest state

15.   An increase in potassium blood levels is known as:

   a.   Hypernatremia

   b.   Hypokalemia

   c.   Hypercalcemia

   d.   Hyperkalemia

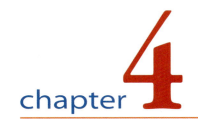

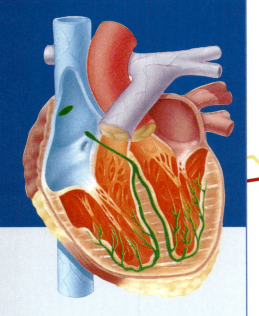

The Electrical Conduction System

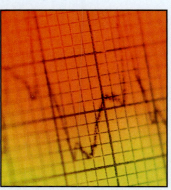

g. Bundle branches

h. Purkinje network

➤ Relate the normal path of an impulse traveling through the electrical conduction system

INTRODUCTION

The heart's pacing, or conduction, system is responsible for the electrical activity that controls each normal heartbeat. This unique system consists of specialized cells and fibers that are collectively known as nodes or bundles. These nodes and bundles are relatively small and are located primarily beneath the endocardium (the innermost lining of the chambers of the heart). Specialized parts of this system are capable of initiating electrical activity automatically and can act as pacemakers for the heart. (See Figure 4–1 and Table 4–1.)

A thorough understanding of the electrical conduction system of the heart is an essential component of learning and understanding an EKG strip.

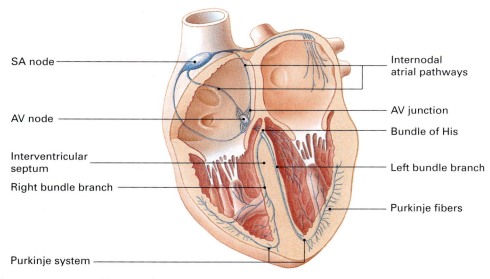

SA node

Internodal atrial pathways

AV node

AV junction

Bundle of His

Interventricular septum

Right bundle branch

Left bundle branch

Purkinje fibers

Purkinje system

Figure 4–1. Cardiac conduction system

Table 4–1

Review of the electrical conduction system of the heart				
SA Node	**Internodal Pathways**	**AV Junction, AV Node, and Bundle**	**Bundle Branches**	**Purkinje Network**
Firing rate 60–100 bpm	Transfer impulse from the SA node throughout the atria to the AV junction	Slows impulse intrinsic firing rate of 40–60 bpm	Two main branches (left and right) transmit impulse to ventricles	Spreads impulse throughout the ventricles; intrinsic firing rate 20–40 bpm

While it is important to note that the EKG strip itself is representative of only the electrical activity of the heart, the student must also understand that the clinician cannot determine the mechanical activity of a patient's heart by merely looking at an EKG strip.

In order to begin to determine that an EKG strip is "abnormal," the student must first understand the normal parameters for the graphic representation of the electrical activity of the heart. It is to that end that this chapter is presented. In this chapter, you will learn where the pacemakers and conducting fibers are located, as well as how they function during a normal heartbeat.

SA NODE

The sinoatrial (SA) node is located in the upper posterior portion of the right atrial wall of the heart, near the opening of the superior vena cava. The node is made up of a cluster of hundreds of cells: a knot of modified heart muscle. This cluster is capable of generating impulses that travel throughout the muscle fibers of both atria, resulting in depolarization. The SA node primarily receives its blood supply from the SA artery. The SA artery is a branch of the right coronary artery in approximately 60–70 percent of the population. However, in approximately 30–40 percent of the population, the circumflex artery supplies blood to the SA node.

The **SA node** is commonly referred to as the primary pacemaker of the heart because it normally depolarizes more rapidly than any other part of the conduction system. The normal range, or firing rate, of the heart's primary pacemaker (the SA node) is 60 to 100 beats per minute (bpm).

If, for any of a variety of reasons, the dominant pacemaker fails to fire within the normal range, another group of specialized tissues, such as the atrioventricular tissue or the Purkinje network of fibers, will assume the duties of the pacemaker. These backup pacemakers are arranged in a waterfall fashion. Depolarization and resultant myocardial contraction occur as the impulse leaves the SA node and travels further down the path of the electrical conduction system.

INTERNODAL PATHWAYS

Three **internodal tracts** or pathways receive the electrical impulse as it leaves the SA node. These tracts distribute the electrical impulse throughout the atria and transmit the impulse from the SA node to the AV node. The internodal tracts consist of anterior, middle, and posterior divisions.

BACHMANN'S BUNDLE

Bachmann's bundle is a group of interatrial fibers contained in the left atrium. It is a subdivision of the anterior internodal tract. This specialized group of cardiac fibers conducts electrical activity from the SA node to the left atrium.

AV NODE

The **atrioventricular (AV) node** is located on the floor of the right atrium near the opening of the coronary sinus and just above the tricuspid valve. At the level of the AV node, the electrical activity is delayed approximately 0.05 second. This delay allows for atrial

SA node commonly referred to as the primary pacemaker of the heart because it normally depolarizes more rapidly than any other part of the conduction system

internodal tracts distribute the electrical impulse throughout the atria and transmit the impulse from the SA node to the AV node

Bachmann's bundle a subdivision of the anterior internodal tract, conducts electrical activity from the SA node to the left atrium

atrioventricular (AV) node located on the floor of the right atrium near the opening of the coronary sinus and just above the tricuspid valve; at the level of the AV node, the electrical activity is delayed approximately 0.05 second

contraction and a more complete filling of the ventricles. The AV node includes three regions: the AV junctional tissue between the atria and node, the nodal area, and the AV junctional tissue between the node and the bundle of His. In the normal heart, the AV node is the only pathway for conduction of atrial electrical impulses to the ventricles.

AV JUNCTION

The region where the AV node joins the bundle of His is called the **AV junction**. Similar to the SA node, the AV junctional tissue contains fibers that can depolarize spontaneously, forming an electrical impulse that can spread to the heart chambers. Therefore, if the SA node fails or slows below its normal range, the AV junctional tissues can initiate electrical activity and thus assume the role of a secondary pacemaker.

AV junction the region where the AV node joins the bundle of His

BUNDLE OF HIS

The conduction pathway that leads out of the AV node was described by a German physician, Wilhelm His, in 1893 and has subsequently been referred to as the **bundle of His.** The bundle of His is also referred to as the atrioventricular bundle or the common bundle. It is approximately 15 millimeters long and lies at the top of the interventricular septum, the wall between the right and left ventricles.

 The bundle of His is also traditionally referred to as the *common bundle*. This bundle of specialized cells contains pacemaker cells that have the ability to self-initiate electrical activity at an intrinsic firing rate of 40 to 60 beats per minute.

bundle of His the conduction pathway that leads out of the AV node and is also traditionally referred to as the *common bundle*

BUNDLE BRANCHES

The bundle of His divides into two main branches at the top of the interventricular septum. These branches are the right bundle branch and the left bundle branch. The primary function of the bundle branches is to conduct electrical activity from the bundle of His down to the Purkinje network. A long, thin structure lying beneath the endocardium, the right bundle branch runs down the right side of the interventricular septum and terminates at the papillary muscles in the right ventricle. This bundle branch functions to carry electrical impulses to the right ventricle.

 Shorter than the right bundle branch, the left bundle branch divides into pathways that spread from the left side of the interventricular septum and throughout the left ventricle. The two main divisions of the left bundle branch are called *fascicles.* The anterior fascicle carries electrical impulses to the anterior wall of the left ventricle, and the posterior fascicle spreads the impulses to the posterior ventricular wall. The bundle branches continue to divide until they finally terminate in the Purkinje fibers.

bundle branches two main branches, the right bundle branch and the left bundle branch, conduct electrical activity from the bundle of His down to the Purkinje network

PURKINJE'S NETWORK

Bundle branches lead to a network of small conduction fibers that spread throughout the ventricles. These fibers were first described in 1787 by Johannes E. Purkinje, a Czechoslovakian physiologist. This network of fibers carries electrical impulses directly to ventricular muscle cells. The fibers that connect with Purkinje's fibers start in the atrioventricular node in the right atrium of the heart.

Purkinje's Network a network of fibers that carries electrical impulses directly to ventricular muscle cells

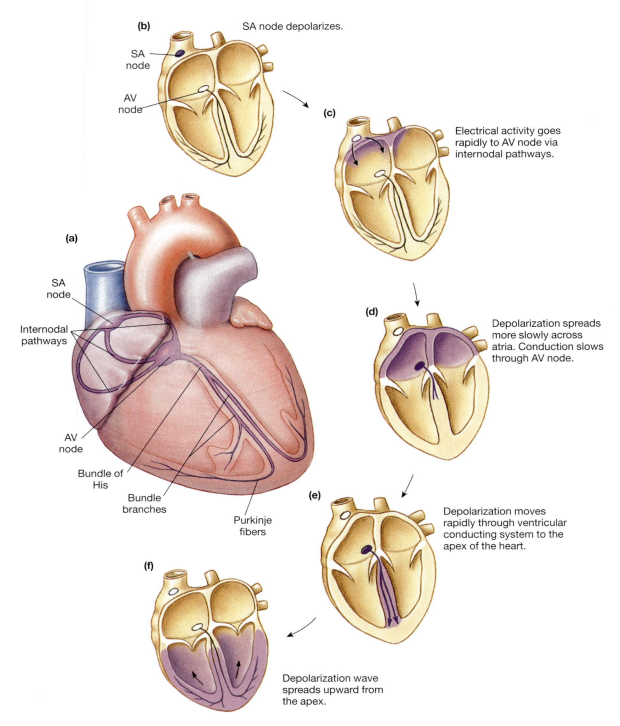

(b) SA node depolarizes.

SA node

AV node

(c) Electrical activity goes rapidly to AV node via internodal pathways.

(a)

SA node

Internodal pathways

AV node

Bundle of His

Bundle branches

Purkinje fibers

(d) Depolarization spreads more slowly across atria. Conduction slows through AV node.

(e) Depolarization moves rapidly through ventricular conducting system to the apex of the heart.

(f) Depolarization wave spreads upward from the apex.

Figure 4–2.   Electrical conduction system in the heart

Purkinje's network can be identified only with the aid of a microscope, but these fibers are larger in diameter than ordinary cardiac muscle fibers. Ventricular contraction is facilitated by the rapid spread of the electrical impulse through the left and right bundle branches and Purkinje fibers, into the ventricular muscle. Purkinje's network fibers possess the intrinsic ability to serve as a pacemaker. The firing rate of the Purkinje pacemaker fibers is normally within the range of 20 to 40 beats per minute.

SUMMARY

A thorough understanding of the heart's normal electrical conduction system is vital to your understanding of the various heart rhythms. In order to understand the causes of dysrhythmias, it is imperative that you have a working knowledge of the underlying concepts of normal sinus rhythm. As you now understand, the electrical impulse arises in the SA node and terminates in the Purkinje network.

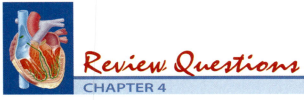

Review Questions

CHAPTER 4

1. The sinoatrial node is located in the:
    a. Right atrium
    b. Right ventricle
    c. Purkinje fiber tract
    d. Atrioventricular septum

2. The AV node is located in the:
    a. Right atrium
    b. Left ventricle
    c. Purkinje fiber tract
    d. Atrioventricular septum

3. The intrinsic firing rate of the AV junction is _____ bpm.
    a. 15–20
    b. 25–35
    c. 35–45
    d. 40–60

4. The intrinsic firing rate of the SA node is _____ bpm.
    a. 20–60
    b. 40–80
    c. 60–100
    d. 80–100

5. The electrocardiogram is used to:
    a. Determine pulse rate
    b. Detect valvular dysfunction
    c. Evaluate electrical activity in the heart
    d. Determine whether the heart is beating

6. The normal conduction pattern of the heart follows the sequence:
    1. SA node
    2. Purkinje fibers
    3. Bundle of His
    4. AV node

    5. Bundle branches

    6. Internodal pathways

  a. 1, 2, 3, 5, 6, 4

  b. 1, 6, 4, 3, 5, 2

  c. 1, 6, 4, 2, 3, 5

  d. 6, 1, 5, 4, 3, 2

7. The intrinsic firing rate of the Purkinje network is _____ bpm.

  a. 60–80

  b. 40–60

  c. 20–40

  d. 10–20

8. The SA node receives its blood supply primarily from the:

  a. Coronary artery

  b. Great cardiac vein

  c. SA artery

  d. Aorta

9. _____ internodal tracts or pathways receive the electrical impulse as it leaves the SA node. These tracts distribute the electrical impulse throughout the atria and transmit the impulse from the SA node to the AV node.

  a. Two

  b. Three

  c. Four

  d. Five

10. What is the specialized group of cardiac fibers conducting electrical activity from the SA node to the left atrium?

  a. Purkinje network

  b. Bundle of His

  c. Bachmann's bundle

  d. Intercalated disks

11. The interventricular septum is the wall between the:

  a. Right and left atrium

  b. Right and left ventricle

  c. Inferior and superior chambers

  d. Inferior and superior vena cavae

12. Purkinje's network fibers can be identified only with the aid of a microscope.

  a. True

  b. False

INTRODUCTION

The medical use of the electrocardiogram dates back to less than a century ago, around the year 1900. The equipment used at that time was large, cumbersome and certainly not appropriate for use in small or confined spaces. Modern technology has brought us very far in the past 100 years, to the point where every Emergency Department and prehospital advanced life support unit has equipment suitable for obtaining an EKG on a patient whenever and wherever indicated. The most significant lesson that you will learn while traveling through this textbook centers not on the EKG tracing, but on the clinical picture of your patient. You must continually ask yourself "How is this rhythm clinically significant to the patient?" Regardless of the pattern observed on the oscilloscope, your patient's condition is and must be, your primary concern. Keep this important fact in mind, and your patient's best interest will always be served.

THE ELECTROCARDIOGRAM

electrocardiogram graphic representation of the electrical activity of the heart

electrocardiograph machine used to record the electrocardiogram

The **electrocardiogram** (EKG or ECG—both abbreviations are acceptable) is commonly defined as a graphic representation of the electrical activity of the heart. (See Figure 5–1.) The machine used to record the electrocardiogram is called an **electrocardiograph,** or more simply an EKG machine.

While EKG analysis serves as a useful diagnostic tool, the health care professional must be cognizant of the fact that the EKG is a graphic tracing of the **electrical activity** of the heart but not the **mechanical activity.** Thus, while much worthwhile information can be obtained from an EKG strip, there is certain valuable information that cannot be gleaned from the strip alone.

Table 5–1 depicts the information which can and that which cannot be obtained from the analysis of an EKG strip.

ELECTRICAL BASIS OF THE EKG

In Chapter 4, we explored the components and functions of the heart's electrical conduction system. On the basis of that knowledge, we should understand that the heart generates electrical activity in the body; thus the body can be thought of as a major conductor of electrical activity. This electrical activity can be sensed by electrodes placed on the skin surface and can be recorded in the form of an electrocardiogram. Cardiac monitors depict the heart's electrical impulses as patterns of waves on the monitor screen or oscilloscope. Because electrical impulses present on the skin surface are of very low voltage, the impulses must be amplified by the EKG machine. The printed record of the electrical activity of the heart is called a **rhythm strip** or an **EKG strip** (Figure 5–2).

rhythm strip or EKG strip the printed record of the electrical activity of the heart

electrode an adhesive pad that contains conductive gel and is designed to be attached to the patient's skin

leads electrodes connected to the monitor or EKG machine by wires

EKG LEADS

As we discussed earlier in this chapter, the cardiac monitor receives electrical impulses from the patient's heart through electrodes placed on particular areas of the body. An **electrode** is an adhesive pad that contains conductive gel and is designed to be attached to the patient's skin. The electrodes are then connected to the monitor or EKG machine by wires called **leads.** These wires are generally color-coded in order to be user-friendly.

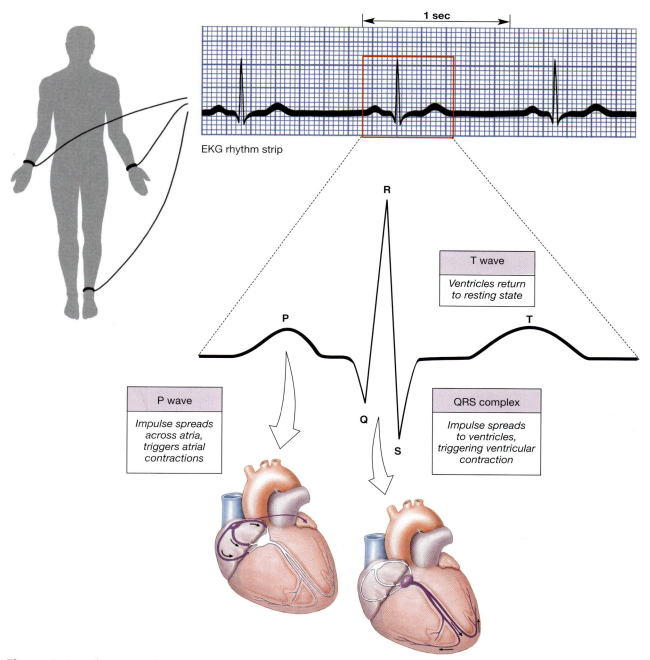

Figure 5–1.   Electrocardiogram

In EKG monitoring, the term **Lead** is sometimes used in two different contexts. We use the other meaning of the term when speaking of a pair of electrodes: chest Lead I, II, MCL, etc. In this usage, the term is generally capitalized.

For the monitor or EKG machine to receive a clear picture of the electrical impulses generated by the heart's electrical conduction system, there must be a positive, a negative, and a ground lead. The ground lead serves to minimize outside electrical interference. The exact portion of the heart being visualized depends, in large part, on the placement of electrodes.

Lead a pair of electrodes such as chest Lead I, II, MCL

Table 5–1

Information obtainable from EKG strip analysis:		
Heart rate	Yes	
Rhythm or regularity	Yes	
Impulse conduction time intervals	Yes	
Abnormal conduction pathways	Yes	
Pumping action		No
Cardiac output		No
Blood pressure		No
Cardiac muscle hypertrophy		No

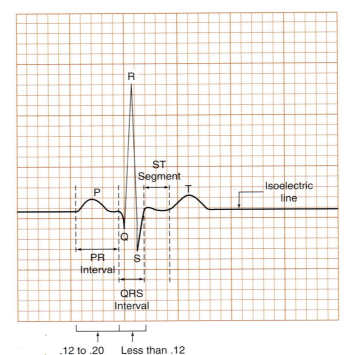

Figure 5–2. EKG

It may be helpful to envision the heart as an object placed on a pedestal around which a person can move while taking photographs (different views) from all angles. This analogy would describe the 12-lead EKG, whereas only one snapshot or view of the heart would represent the 3-lead EKG. The 12-lead EKG is commonly used in hospitals and clinics; the 3-lead EKG is typically used in the field. It should be noted that some of the newer monitors require a fourth lead, which represents the right leg. In some areas of the country, 12-lead EKGs are being used regularly to aid in screening patients who are potential candidates for fibrinolytic (thrombolytic) therapy. It is important to note that the 3-lead EKG is sufficient for detecting life-threatening **dysrhythmias**.

Lead II and the MCL (modified chest lead) are most commonly used for cardiac monitoring because of their ability to visualize P waves. Chest Leads I, II, and III are known as **bipolar leads,** which means that these leads have one positive electrode and one negative electrode. Bipolar leads are sometimes referred to as limb leads. Table 5–2

dysrhythmias
abnormal rhythms

bipolar leads
have one positive electrode and one negative electrode

Table 5–2

Placement of bipolar leads		
Lead	**Positive Electrode**	**Negative Electrode**
I	Left arm	Right arm
II	Left leg	Right arm
III	Left leg	Left arm

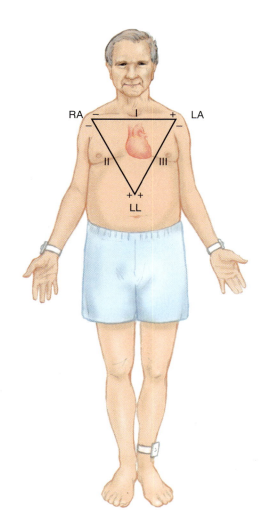

Figure 5–3.   Einthoven's triangle

represents the placement of electrodes of the three bipolar leads on certain areas of the body.

An imaginary inverted triangle is formed around the heart by proper placement of the bipolar leads. This triangle is referred to as Einthoven's triangle (Figure 5–3). The top of the triangle is formed by Lead I, the right side of the triangle is formed by Lead II, and the left side of the triangle is formed by Lead III. Each lead represents a different look at or view of the heart. For the sake of consistency, chest Lead II will be used throughout this textbook, except where otherwise designated.

EKG GRAPH PAPER

Electrocardiographic paper (Figure 5–4) is arranged as a series of horizontal and vertical lines printed on graph paper and provides a printed record of cardiac electrical activity. This paper is standardized to allow for consistency in analyzing EKG rhythm strips. EKG paper leaves the machine at a constant speed of 25 millimeters per second (mm/s).

Both time and amplitude (or voltage) are measured on graph paper. Time is measured on the horizontal line; amplitude or voltage is measured on the vertical line. The vertical axis reflects millivolts (mV); two large squares = 1 mV. EKG graph paper is divided into small squares, each of which is 1 millimeter (mm) in height and width and represents a time interval of 0.04 second. Darker lines further divide the paper every fifth square, both vertically and horizontally. Each of these large squares measures 5 millimeters in height and 5 millimeters in width and represents a time interval of 0.20 second. There are five small squares in each large square. Therefore 5 small squares × 0.04 second = 0.20 second. The squares on the EKG paper represent the measurement of the length of time required for the electrical impulse to traverse a specific part of the heart. Proper interpretation of EKG rhythms is dependent in part, on the understanding of the time increments as represented on EKG paper (Figure 5–4).

EKG WAVEFORMS

A wave or waveform recorded on an EKG strip refers to movement away from the baseline, or isoelectric line, and is represented as a positive deflection (above the isoelectric line) or as a negative deflection (below the isoelectric line). The **baseline** is the straight line seen on an EKG strip; it represents the beginning and end point of all waves.

As the electrical impulse leaves the SA node, waveforms are produced on the graph paper. One complete cardiac cycle is represented on graph paper by five major waves: the P wave; the Q, R, and S waves (normally referred to as the QRS complex); and the T wave.

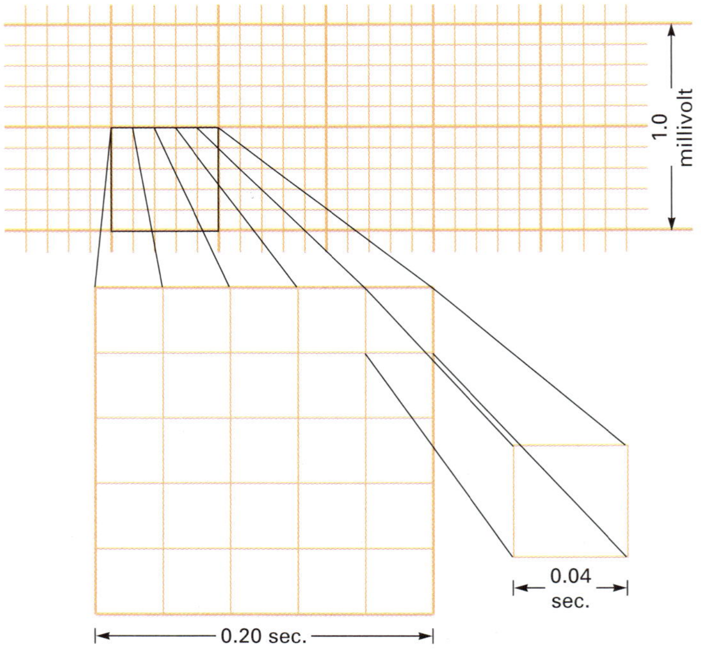

EKG waveforms
a wave or waveform recorded on an EKG strip refers to movement away from the baseline or isoelectric line and is represented as a positive deflection (above the isoelectric line) or as a negative deflection (below the isoelectric line)

baseline the straight line seen on an EKG strip; it represents the beginning and end point of all waves

Figure 5–4. EKG paper and markings

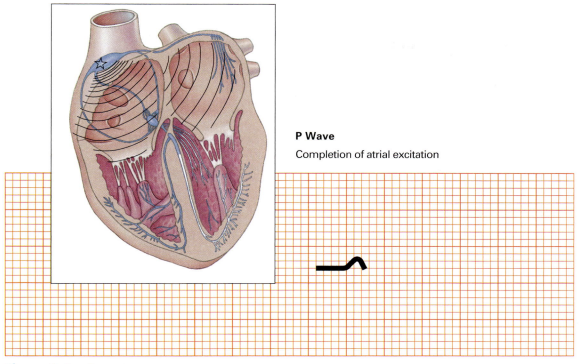

P Wave

Completion of atrial excitation

Figure 5–5.   P wave

P wave

As we discussed in Chapter 4, the SA node fires first during a normal cardiac cycle. This "firing" event sends the electrical impulse outward to stimulate both atria and manifests as the P wave (Figure 5–5). When observed on a Lead II EKG strip, the **P wave** is a smooth, rounded upward deflection. The P wave represents depolarization of the left and right atria and is approximately 0.10 second in length.

P wave represents depolarization of the left and right atria

PR interval

The **PR interval** (Figure 5–6), sometimes abbreviated PRI, represents the time interval necessary for the impulse to travel from the SA node through the internodal pathways in the atria and downward to the ventricles. In simpler terms, the PRI is said to represent the distance from the beginning of the P wave to the beginning of the QRS complex. The normal PR interval is measured as 3–5 small squares of the EKG graph paper and is 0.12–0.20 second in length.

PR interval represents the time interval necessary for the impulse to travel from the SA node through the internodal pathways in the atria and downward to the ventricles

QRS complex

The **QRS complex** (Figure 5–7) consists of the Q, R, and S waves and represents the conduction of the electrical impulse from the bundle of His throughout the ventricular muscle, or ventricular depolarization. The Q wave is seen as the first downward deflection following the PRI. The R wave is the first upward deflection of the QRS complex and is normally the largest deflection seen in chest Leads I and II. Immediately following the R wave, there is a downward deflection, which is called the S wave.

The QRS complex is measured from the beginning of the Q wave to the point where the S wave meets the baseline. Normally, the QRS complex measures less than 0.12 second

QRS complex consists of the Q, R, and S waves and represents the conduction of the electrical impulse from the bundle of His throughout the ventricular muscle, or ventricular depolarization

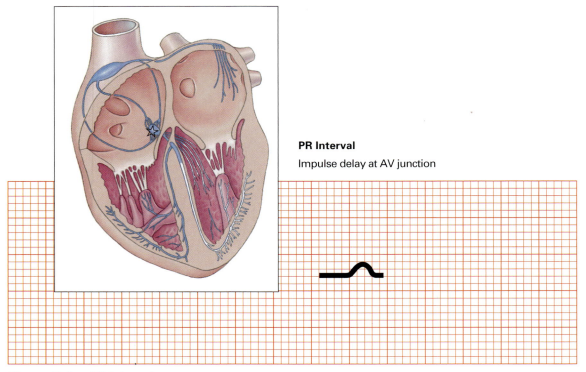

PR Interval

Impulse delay at AV junction

Figure 5–6. PR interval

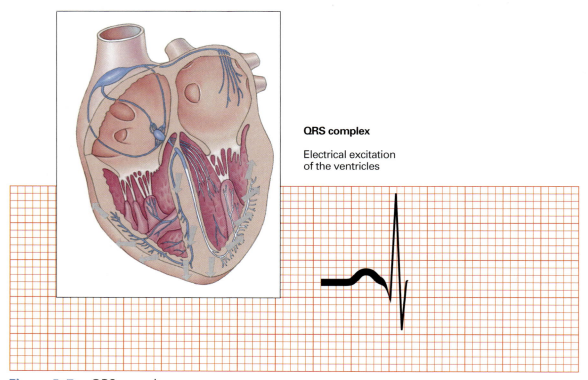

QRS complex

Electrical excitation
of the ventricles

Figure 5–7. QRS complex

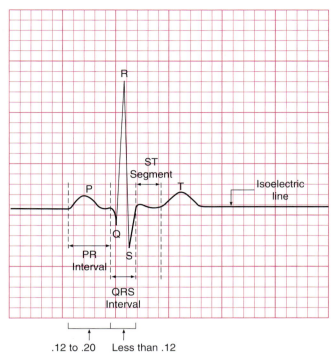

Figure 5–8. EKG waveforms

or less than three small squares on EKG graph paper. It should be noted that the shape of the QRS complex will vary from individual to individual and not all three waves are necessarily present.

ST segment

The time interval during which the ventricles are depolarized and ventricular repolarization begins is called the **ST segment**. (See Figure 5–8.) Normally the ST segment is isoelectric, or consistent with the baseline. In certain cardiac disease processes, the ST segment may be elevated or depressed due to ischemia, infarction, or both. Elevation of the ST segment is one of the major EKG changes appreciated in an acute myocardial infarction.

ST segment the time interval during which the ventricles are depolarized and ventricular repolarization begins

T wave

Following the ST segment is the **T wave** (Figure 5–9), which represents ventricular repolarization. The T wave is normally seen as a slightly asymmetrical, slightly rounded, positive deflection. Recall now that ventricular repolarization is an electrical event with no associated activity of the ventricular musculature. The T wave is often referred to as the **resting phase** of the cardiac cycle.

Recall also that the refractory periods, both absolute and relative, are in place during the EKG representation of the T wave and thus the heart may be vulnerable to strong impulses which may lead to ventricular dysrhythmias. The T wave may be either elevated or depressed in the presence of current or previous cardiac ischemia. Normally one complete cardiac cycle is represented by the P-QRS-T pattern.

T wave represents ventricular repolarization and follows the ST segment

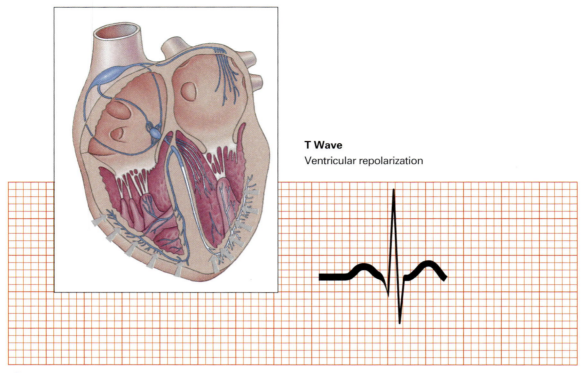

T Wave
Ventricular repolarization

Figure 5–9. T wave

Table 5–3

Summary of EKG waveforms and correlating cardiac events	
P Wave Represents	Atrial Depolarization
QRS complex represents	Ventricular depolarization; atrial repolarization
T wave represents	Ventricular repolarization

SUMMARY

Now that we have discussed the components of the electrocardiogram, let me remind you that it is imperative always, at all times, to **observe and treat the patient on the basis of his or her clinical presentation, regardless of the rhythm being observed on the oscilloscope!** Always remember to ask yourself, "How is this rhythm clinically significant to my patient?"

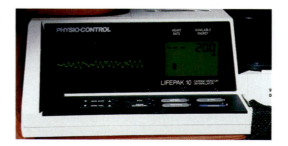

Figure 5–10. Cardiac monitor

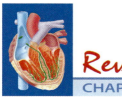

Review Questions

1. Ventricular diastole refers to ventricular:
    a. Contraction
    b. Relaxation
    c. Filling time
    d. Pressure ratio

2. The electrocardiogram is used to:
    a. Determine cardiac output
    b. Detect valvular dysfunction
    c. Evaluate electrical activity in the heart
    d. Detect left to right conduction disorders

3. The PR interval should normally be _____ second or smaller.
    a. 0.10
    b. 0.12
    c. 0.08
    d. 0.20

4. The QRS interval should normally be _____ second or smaller.
    a. 0.20
    b. 0.12
    c. 0.18
    d. 0.36

5. The QRS complex is produced when:
    a. The ventricles repolarize
    b. The ventricles depolarize
    c. The ventricles contract
    d. Both b and c

6. The normal conduction pattern of the heart follows which sequence?
    1. SA node
    2. Purkinje fibers
    3. Bundle of His
    4. AV node
    5. Bundle branches
    6. Internodal pathways

a. 1, 5, 2, 4, 6, 3

b. 1, 6, 4, 3, 5, 2

c. 1, 4, 3, 6, 5, 2

d. 1, 2, 3, 4, 5, 6

7. The T wave on the EKG strip represents:

a. Rest period

b. Bundle of His

c. Atrial contraction

d. Ventricular contraction

8. The coronary circulation has how many main arteries?

a. Two

b. Six

c. Four

d. Eight

9. When interpreting dysrhythmias, the health care provider should remember that the most important key is the:

a. PR interval

b. Rate and rhythm

c. Presence of dysrhythmias

d. Patient's clinical appearance

10. A graphic record of the electrical activity of the heart is an:

a. Echocardiogram

b. Electrocardiogram

c. Encephalogram

d. Radiogram

11. While EKG analysis serves as a useful diagnostic tool, the health care professional must be cognizant of the fact that the EKG is a graphic tracing of the electrical activity of the heart but not the mechanical activity.

a. True

b. False

12. The ground lead serves to minimize outside electrical interference.

a. True

b. False

13. The exact portion of the heart being visualized depends, in large part, on the placement of the:

a. Patient

b. Paddles

c. Electrodes

d. Oscilloscope

14. Lead II is most commonly used for cardiac monitoring because of its ability to visualize _____ waves.

    a. P

    b. Q

    c. R

    d. T

15. _____ leads are those that have one positive electrode and one negative electrode.

    a. Bipolar

    b. Unipolar

    c. Multipolar

    d. Tripolar

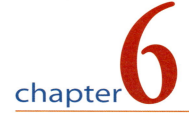

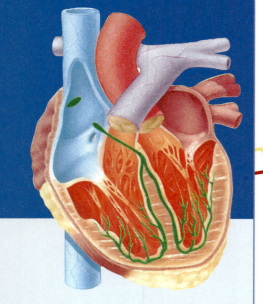

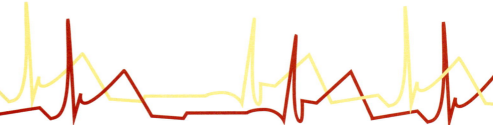

Interpretation of an EKG Strip

objectives

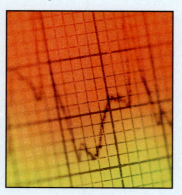

Upon completion of this chapter, the student will be able to:

➤ Describe the basic approach to interpretation of EKG strips

➤ Explain the five steps used in interpretation of EKG strips

➤ Explain how to calculate heart rate, given a 6-second strip

➤ Name four causes of artifact

INTRODUCTION

This is the most important chapter in this textbook! Why would I make such an emphatic statement? Simply because it's true. The preceding chapters were essential building blocks leading up to this chapter, and the subsequent chapters will focus on application of the rules mastered in this chapter. Therefore, this chapter is critical to your understanding of proper interpretation of an EKG rhythm strip. For many years now, I have explained to students that the key to learning, interpreting, and—most importantly—*understanding* dysrhythmias is a systematic approach, which must be used each and every time a strip is analyzed.

Now, let's be honest here. Do I really expect you to believe that all paramedics—even the ones who have been "street medics" for twenty years—always apply this five-step systematic approach for every strip they see? Well, no, not exactly. However, you are utilizing this book because you wish to learn how to interpret dysrhythmias effortlessly. Keep in mind that, while learning this skill, memorization will *not* suffice. You must learn and apply this systematic approach to EKG analysis. When you look at a strip, think about and apply these five steps, and you should be successful in mastering the art of EKG analysis.

GENERAL RULES

Here are a few basic rules that will assist you in your quest to correctly identify heart rhythms.

1. **First and most important, look at your patient!** What is the patient's clinical picture, and how is it significant to the rhythm noted on the monitor?
2. Read EVERY strip from left to right, starting at the beginning of the strip.
3. Apply the five-step systematic approach that you will learn in this chapter.
4. Avoid shortcuts and assumptions. A quick glance at a strip will often lead to an incorrect interpretation.
5. Ask and answer each question in the five-step approach in the order that it is presented here. This is important for consistency.
6. You must master the accepted limits, or parameters, for each dysrhythmia and then apply them to each of the five steps when analyzing the strip.

THE FIVE-STEP APPROACH

There are several appropriate formats for EKG interpretation. The format that I have chosen follows a logical sequence in that we discuss EKG interpretation first on the basis of heart rate and rhythm, and then by analysis of graphic representations of activities as they occur in the electrical conduction system of the heart.

This five-step approach, in order of application, includes analysis of the following:

1. **Step 1:** Heart rate
2. **Step 2:** Heart rhythm
3. **Step 3:** P wave
4. **Step 4:** PR interval
5. **Step 5:** QRS complex

EKG interpretation is more easily accomplished if each step is examined using this approach with each strip. Remember: a quick glance can be deceiving.

Step 1: Heart rate

heart rate the number of electrical impulses conducted through the myocardium in 60 seconds

Heart rate can be defined as the number of electrical impulses (as represented by PQRST complexes) conducted through the myocardium in 60 seconds (1 minute). This analysis should be your first step in the interpretation of an EKG strip. When calculating heart rate, we are usually referring to the **ventricular** heart rate. However, it is appropriate in certain strips to calculate both the atrial heart rate and the ventricular heart rate.

Simply stated, atrial heart rate can be determined by counting the number of P waves noted; ventricular heart rate is determined by counting the number of QRS complexes. If the atrial and ventricular heart rates are dissimilar, it is very important that you calculate both.

Recall now that the SA node discharges impulses at a rate of 60–100 times per minute. Therefore, a "normal" heart rate will be noted if the rate is calculated within a range of 60 to 100 beats per minute (bpm). If the rate is noted to be less than 60 bpm, we refer to it as **bradycardia**. In contrast, if the heart rate is greater than 100 bpm, the correct term is **tachycardia**. It is important to note here that these numbers are simply normal boundaries (sometimes called parameters) to which we adhere when analyzing heart rate.

bradycardia
heart rate of less than 60 bpm

tachycardia heart rate greater than 100 bpm

Keep in mind that your patient's clinical picture is critical to proper assessment and management. In other words, if your patient's heart rate is 58 bpm, he or she is *technically* bradycardic, on the basis of "normal" parameters. The patient's clinical picture, however, may indicate no evidence of compromise. Remember to ask yourself this question: **"How is the rhythm significant to the patient's clinical picture?"** Often you will find that the patient with a heart rate of 58 bpm is exhibiting no clinical symptomatology at all.

There are two methods commonly used to determine heart rate by visual examination of an EKG strip. The first and simplest is called the **6-second method** (Figure 6–1). To use this method properly you must first denote a 6-second interval on an EKG strip. Fortunately for us, EKG paper is commonly marked in either 3- or 6-second increments. Simply count the number of QRS complexes that occur within the 6-second interval and then multiply this number by 10. If the graph paper does not have 3- or 6-second marks,

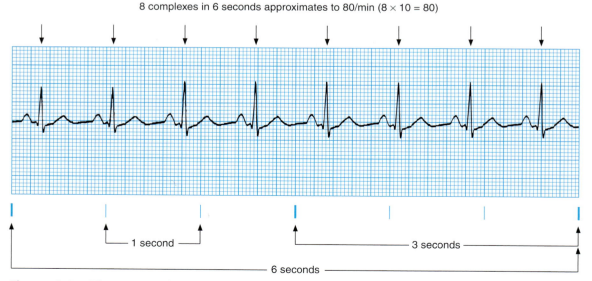

8 complexes in 6 seconds approximates to 80/min (8 × 10 = 80)

Figure 6–1. The 6-second method

you can count the number of R waves in 30 large squares and multiply this number by 10. This will yield a close approximation of the patient's heart rate. This method is effective even when the rhythm is noted to be irregular.

The second common method used to determine heart rate by visual examination of an EKG strip is the **R-R interval** method. This method is most accurate if the heart rhythm is regular; otherwise, it is only an estimation of heart rate. Recall from our discussion of EKG graph paper that there are 300 large boxes in a 60-second or 1-minute strip. With this in mind, you should look for a QRS complex (specifically an R wave) that falls on a heavy line on the strip. Then you should count the number of large boxes between the first R wave and the next R wave. After you determine that number, you divide it into 300. For example, if there are three large boxes between two R to R waves, you would divide 3 into 300 and find that the heart rate is 100 bpm (300 divided by 3 = 100). Apply this method to the strip in Figure 6–2.

Remember that the "normal" heart rate is 60–100 bpm. Below 60 bpm is a slow or bradycardic rate. Greater than 100 bpm is considered a fast or tachycardic rate. Heart rates can vary depending on many factors, including the general health of your patient, as well as stress levels, strenuous exercise, or myocardial compromise. Again, you must constantly assess your patient while assessing his or her EKG strip.

Step 2: Heart rhythm

Now we are ready to move on to step 2 in the systematic approach to EKG analysis. Step 2 involves evaluating the rhythm of the heart. The term **heart rhythm** can be defined as the sequential beating of the heart as a result of the generation of electrical impulses. Synonyms for rhythm include pattern, guide, model, order, and design. Thus we can see that calculating the heart rhythm involves establishing a pattern of QRS complex occurrence. Calculations of heart rhythms are classified as either regular or irregular.

Normally, the heart's rhythm is regular. To determine whether the ventricular rhythm is regular, you should measure the intervals between R to R waves. To determine whether the atrial rhythm is regular, you should measure the intervals between P to P waves. If the intervals vary by less than 0.06 second (or 1.5 small squares), we can consider the rhythm regular. If, however, the intervals are variable by greater than 0.06 second, the rhythm is considered irregular.

It may be helpful to use EKG calipers when you begin to analyze EKG rhythms. If calipers are not available, you may also measure intervals by making marks on a piece of paper placed on the EKG strip just below the peak of the R wave. After marking the area where each R wave occurred, look at the marks on your paper to identify a pattern. Then measure the distance between the marks with a ruler. If the

heart rhythm the sequential beating of the heart as a result of the generation of electrical impulses

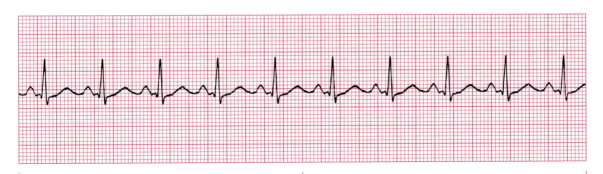

Figure 6–2.   NSR strip with rate of 100

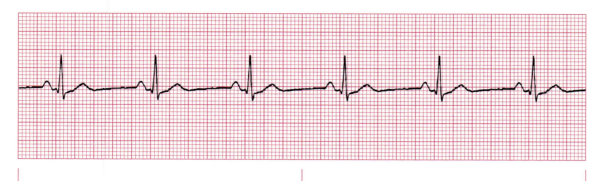

Figure 6–3.   Practice strips for rate and rhythm analysis

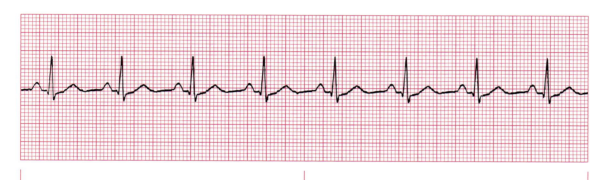

Figure 6–4.   Practice strips for rate and rhythm analysis

marks are relatively equal distances apart, the rhythm is noted to be regular. If the distance between the marks varies noticeably, then the rhythm is probably irregular. Alterations of respiratory rate and depth may produce slight variations in heart rhythms.

Rhythms that are found to be irregular can be further classified as:

a. *Regularly irregular* - irregular rhythms that occur in a pattern.
b. *Occasionally irregular* - intervals of only one or two R-Rs are uneven.
c. *Irregularly irregular* - R-R intervals exhibit no similarity.

Regardless of whether the rhythm is regular or irregular, always remember to ask yourself the all-important question, **"How is this rhythm clinically significant to my patient?"**

Before moving on to step 3, take a moment to review steps 1 and 2. Now look at the two strips in Figures 6–3 and 6–4 and calculate the rate and rhythm of each one. After you think you have the answers, ask your instructor or tutor to verify your answers.

Step 3: The P wave

P waves
depolarization of the atria

First, let's recall the events that must occur to cause the formation of **P waves** on an EKG strip. We learned in Chapter 5 that the P wave is produced when the right and left atria depolarize. Depolarization of the atria is produced when an electrical impulse spreads throughout the atria via the internodal pathways. The P wave is noted as the first deviation from the isoelectric line on the EKG strip and should always be rounded and upright (positive) in chest Lead II. If the P wave is not upright in Lead II, you are not looking at a sinus rhythm (i.e., a rhythm originating in the SA node).

There are five questions that should be asked in evaluating P waves:

1. Are P waves present?
2. Are the P waves occurring regularly?
3. Is there one P wave present for each QRS complex present?
4. Are the P waves smooth, rounded, and upright in appearance, or are they inverted?
5. Do all the P waves look similar?

Recall now that the sinoatrial (SA) node is the primary pacemaker of the heart and is located in the right atrium. If the SA node is pacing or firing at regular intervals, the P waves will also follow at regular intervals. This pattern would then be referred to as a **sinus rhythm.** In this text, the heart rhythms will be referred to according to their points of origin.

Step 4: The PR interval

The **PR interval** measures the time intervals from the onset of atrial contraction to the onset of ventricular contraction, or the time necessary for the electrical impulse to be conducted through the atria and the AV node. Although this component is called the PR interval, it actually includes the entire P wave. The PR interval is measured from the onset (beginning) of the P wave to the onset of the Q wave of the QRS complex.

PR interval measures the time intervals from the onset of atrial contraction to the onset of ventricular contraction

The normal length of the PR interval is 0.12–0.20 second (three to five small squares). The PR interval should be constant across the EKG strip in order to be considered "within normal limits." If the PR interval is shortened (less than 0.12 second), this may be an indication that the usual progression of the impulse was outside the normal route. Prolonged PR intervals (greater than 0.20 second) may indicate a delay in the electrical conduction pathway or an AV block.

There are three questions that should be asked when evaluating PR intervals:

1. Are PR intervals greater than 0.20 second?
2. Are PR intervals less than 0.12 second?
3. Are PR intervals constant across the EKG strip?

Step 5: The QRS complex

The **QRS complex** represents the depolarization (or contraction) of the ventricles. It is important to note whether all QRS complexes look alike, as this similarity will indicate that conduction pathways are invariable and consistent.

QRS complex represents the depolarization (or contraction) of the ventricles

The QRS complex is actually a group of waves, consisting of:

Q wave—the first negative or downward deflection of this large complex. It is a small wave that precedes the R wave. Often the Q wave is not seen.
R wave—the first upward or positive deflection following the P wave. In chest Lead II, the R wave is the tallest waveform noted.
S wave—the sharp, negative (or downward) deflection that follows the R wave.

The overall appearance of the QRS, as well as its width, can provide important information about the electrical conduction system. When the electrical conduction system is functioning normally, the width of the QRS complex will be 0.12 second or less (narrow). This normal or narrow QRS complex indicates that the impulse was not formed in the ventricles and is thus referred to as **supraventricular,** "above the ventricles." Wide

supraventricular above the ventricles

QRS complexes (greater than 0.12 second or three small squares) indicate that the impulse is either of ventricular origin or of supraventricular origin with conduction that is aberrant (deviating from the normal course or pattern).

There are three questions that should be asked in evaluating QRS intervals:

1. Are QRS intervals greater than 0.12 second (wide)? If so, the complex may be ventricular in origin.
2. Are QRS intervals less than 0.12 second (narrow)? If so, the complex is probably supraventricular in origin.
3. Are the QRS complexes similar in appearance across the EKG strip?

It is important to realize that the shape of QRS complexes will vary slightly in individual patients, depending on factors such as heart shape and size, health of the myocardium, and location and placement of electrodes.

ST SEGMENT

ST segment
begins with the end of the QRS complex and ends with the onset of the T wave

The **ST segment** begins with the end of the QRS complex and ends with the onset of the T wave. The normal ST segment is usually consistent with the isoelectric line of the EKG strip. The point where the QRS complex meets the ST segment is commonly referred to as the **J point** (Figure 6–5). If the ST segment is elevated or depressed, myocardial ischemia may be indicated.

J point the point where the QRS complex meets the ST segment

THE T WAVE

T wave produced by ventricular repolarization or relaxation

The **T wave** is produced by ventricular repolarization or relaxation. Recall our discussion of the heart's refractory periods to emphasize the importance of the T wave. T waves are commonly seen as the first upward or positive deflection following the QRS complex.

THE U WAVE

U waves are usually not visible on EKG strips, and their cause or origin is not completely understood. Some cardiovascular physiologists now believe that the U wave may represent Purkinje fiber repolarization. When they can be distinguished, U waves typi-

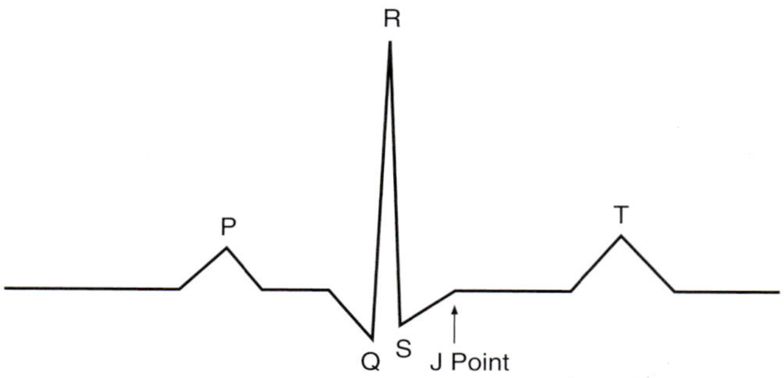

Figure 6–5. J point

cally follow the T wave. The U wave, when present, will appear much smaller than the T wave and will commonly be rounded and upright or positive in deflection.

ARTIFACT

Artifact is defined as EKG waveforms from sources outside the heart. Artifact is interference seen on a monitor or an EKG strip. (See Figure 6–6.) Four common causes of artifact are the following.

artifact EKG waveforms from sources outside the heart

1. *Patient movement* – One type of artifact, called a wandering baseline, may be produced when the patient moves about on the bed or gurney and can usually be corrected when the patient lies still.
2. *Loose or defective electrodes* – When electrodes have lost contact with the patient's skin or when the conductive gel on the electrode has dried, one type of artifact—which may appear as a "fuzzy baseline"—is called 60-cycle interference. This may also result from clammy skin or excessive chest hair. Interference from electrical equipment may also cause 60-cycle interference.
3. *Improper grounding* – Artifact can occur when the patient is in touch with an outside source of electricity, such as a poorly grounded electrical bed; 60-cycle interference may also be caused by improper grounding.
4. *Faulty EKG apparatus* – Broken wires or cables may produce artifact. This is easily corrected by replacing the faulty wires with new ones.

Artifacts can mimic certain lethal dysrhythmias. Therefore, **patient assessment is critical.** Remember that if your patient is lying quietly on the gurney or bed and is engaging in a lively conversation with you regarding his or her past medical history, chances are very good that he or she is not in ventricular fibrillation, regardless of what the monitor shows!

SUMMARY

This is the most important chapter in this textbook, in that you must have a logical, systematic approach to interpreting EKGs. It is imperative that you follow this approach each time you practice EKG analysis, both to increase your confidence as well as to ensure accuracy in interpretation and consequently in your provision of patient care.

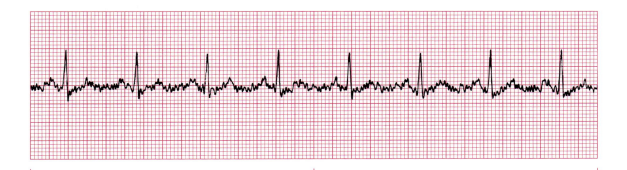

Figure 6–6.   Artifact

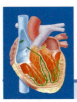

Review Questions

CHAPTER 6

1. When dealing with EKG interpretation, you should always avoid shortcuts and assumptions, because often a quick glance at a strip will lead to an incorrect interpretation.
   a. False
   b. True

2. The intrinsic firing rate of the AV node per minute is: _____ bpm.
   a. 15–25
   b. 25–35
   c. 35–45
   d. 40–60

3. You must master the accepted parameters for each dysrhythmia and then apply those parameters to each of the five steps when analyzing an EKG strip.
   a. True
   b. False

4. The electrocardiogram is used to:
   a. Determine pulse rate
   b. Detect valvular dysfunction
   c. Evaluate electrical activity in the heart
   d. Determine whether the heart is beating

5. The PR interval should normally be _____ second or smaller.
   a. 0.10
   b. 0.12
   c. 0.08
   d. 0.20

6. The QRS interval should normally be _____ second or smaller.
   a. 0.20
   b. 0.12
   c. 0.18
   d. 0.36

7. Artifact is defined as EKG waveforms from sources outside the heart.
   a. True
   b. False

8. Causes of artifact include:
    a. Patient movement
    b. Loose electrodes
    c. Improper grounding
    d. All of the above apply

9. The point at which the QRS complex meets the ST segment is commonly referred to as the:
    a. T point
    b. J point
    c. PRI
    d. S point

10. The term "supraventricular" refers to a stimulus arising above the ventricles.
    a. True
    b. False

11. The T wave on the EKG strip represents:
    a. Rest period
    b. Bundle of His
    c. Atrial contraction
    d. Ventricular contraction

12. When interpreting dysrhythmias, you should remember that the most important key is the:
    a. PR interval
    b. Rate & rhythm
    c. Presence of dysrhythmias
    d. Patient's clinical appearance

13. The health care professional should read EVERY EKG strip from left to right, starting at the beginning of the strip.
    a. True
    b. False

14. The sharp, negative deflection that follows the R wave is called the Q wave.
    a. True
    b. False

15. Heart rhythms are classified as either regular or irregular.
    a. True
    b. False

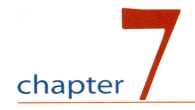

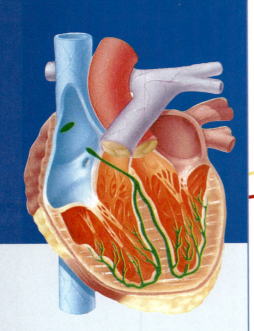

Introducing the Sinus Rhythms

objectives

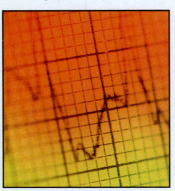

Upon completion of this chapter, the student will be able to:

➤ Discuss the origin of the sinus rhythms

➤ Identify the components of the electrical conduction system of the heart

➤ Identify a normal sinus rhythm, including EKG characteristics

➤ Describe a sinus bradycardia rhythm, including EKG characteristics

➤ Identify a sinus tachycardia rhythm, including EKG characteristics

➤ Describe a sinus dysrhythmia, including EKG characteristics

➤ Describe a sinus arrest rhythm, including EKG characteristics

➤ Discuss the clinical significance of the sinus rhythms

INTRODUCTION

Now the time has come for you to begin to apply the knowledge that you gained from studying Chapters 1–6. You learned in Chapter 6 that you must **always, always** apply the five-step approach to each rhythm strip as you attempt to interpret the rhythm. For the sake of emphasis, let's call this the golden rule of EKG interpretation: **No shortcuts are allowed!**

You will ask yourself five essential questions, and when you decide on the answer to each question, you will be able to interpret the rhythm. In their outstanding book *Advanced Cardiac Life Support,* my colleagues Randall Benner, Gregg Margolis, and Joe Mistovich have pointed out the "red flag" method of analyzing EKG strips: When you find one parameter that falls out of the normal range, it should raise a "red flag" in your thought processes. This method works very well, especially for the novice student. Remember that an abnormal heart rhythm is most commonly referred to as a **dysrhythmia**.

dysrhythmia
abnormal heart rhythm

In this and subsequent chapters, you will be interpreting strips from actual patients as well as strips produced from EKG generators. Remember that rhythm presentations will vary from patient to patient; regardless of the appearance of the waveforms, it is essential that you ask the five questions you have mastered. Only then will you be able to decide which rhythm you are observing. Don't be afraid to ask for help. It takes time and practice to master the art of EKG interpretation.

ORIGIN OF THE SINUS RHYTHMS

As we begin to examine heart rhythms, it is important to remember that rhythms are classified according to the heart structure or structures in which they begin, their **site of origin.** It is also helpful to think about the **name** of each rhythm in order to recall the site of origin of that specific rhythm. Recall now that the sinoatrial (SA) node normally generates impulses at a rate of 60–100 beats per minute (bpm). This characteristic is known as the **inherent** or **intrinsic** rate of the heart's primary pacemaker, the SA node. Thus, rhythms that originate in the SA node are called either sinus rhythms or sinus dysrhythmias.

site of origin
rhythms are classified according to the heart structure or structures in which they begin

COMPONENTS OF THE ELECTRICAL CONDUCTION SYSTEM OF THE HEART

Let's review briefly the components of the electrical conduction system. Normally, the electrical impulse originates in the sinoatrial (SA) node, which is located in the upper right atrium. As the impulse leaves the SA node, it travels through the atria via the internodal pathways. The impulse then reaches the atrioventricular (AV) node, where there is a brief pause. We often consider the AV node the "gatekeeper" to the ventricles. Leaving the AV node, the electrical impulse travels through the right and left bundle branches into and through the Purkinje fibers of the ventricular musculature.

Included in the heart's electrical conduction system are three pacemaker sites. The SA node is the primary pacemaker; the AV node and the Purkinje network are the backup or secondary pacemakers. The SA node is located in the upper right atrium and has an inherent firing rate of 60–100 beats per minute. The AV node is located on the floor of the right atrium and has an intrinsic firing rate of 40–60 beats per minute. The Purkinje fibers are located in the septum and in the ventricles and have an intrinsic firing rate of 20–40 beats per minute. On the basis of your knowledge of the intrinsic firing

normal sinus rhythm the rhythm that occurs when the SA node has generated an impulse that followed the normal pathway of the electrical conduction system and led to atrial and ventricular depolarization

rate of the SA node, what would you expect the rate of a sinus rhythm to be? By this time you may have immediately thought: 60–100 beats per minute! If so, you're on your way. Remember that the first question to ask yourself in the five-step approach is "What is the heart rate?" Now, let's review once more (Tables 7–1 and 7–2).

NORMAL SINUS RHYTHM

In reality, the **only** "normal" rhythm is normal sinus rhythm (NSR). When you ask the questions in the five-step approach, the answers you derive will be and must be within normal limits in order for you to acknowledge that the rhythm you are analyzing is indeed a **normal sinus rhythm.** Although the appearance of the waves can vary, if the answer to all five questions are within normal limits, the rhythm is, quite simply, normal. The SA node has generated an impulse that followed the normal pathway of the electrical conduction system and led to atrial and ventricular depolarization.

The heart rate falls within the range of 60–100 bpm, the atrial and ventricular rhythms are regular, there is a P wave that preceded every QRS complex, all PR intervals range from 0.12 to 0.20 second in length, and the QRS complex is less than 0.12 second. In other words, all five parameters are within normal limits. The rhythm is a normal sinus rhythm (Table 7–3).

Table 7–1

Electrical conduction system pathway

SA node	Internodal pathways	AV node	Bundle of His	Bundle branches	Purkinje network

Table 7–2

Pacemaker sites

SA (sinoatrial) node	Intrinsic rate of 60–100 bpm
AV (atrioventricular) node	Intrinsic rate of 40–60 bpm
Purkinje network	Intrinsic rate of 20–40 bpm

Table 7–3

Normal sinus rhythm

Questions 1–5	Answers
1. What is the rate?	60–100 beats per minute
2. What is the rhythm?	Atrial rhythm regular Ventricular rhythm regular
3. Is there a P wave before each QRS? Are the P waves upright and uniform?	Yes Yes
4. What is the length of the PR interval?	0.12–0.20 second (3–5 small squares)
5. Do all the QRS complexes look alike? What is the length of the QRS complexes?	Yes Less than 0.12 second (3 small squares)

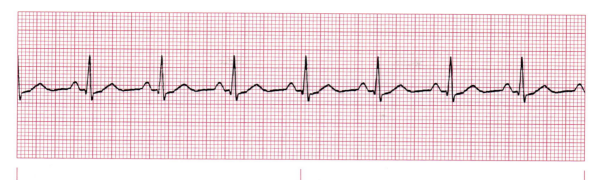

Figure 7–1.   Normal sinus rhythm

Now you should look at the rhythm in Figure 7–1 and slowly, systematically apply each of the five questions, in order to **prove** to yourself that this rhythm is indeed a normal sinus rhythm. **Remember . . . always monitor your patient's condition!**

SINUS BRADYCARDIA RHYTHM

In initial lectures (and just for fun), I often tell students that a normal sinus rhythm has two "first cousins," Sinus bradycardia and Sinus tachycardia. One of those "cousins" will be discussed here now, the other next. At first glance, this rhythm may resemble a normal sinus rhythm, and as a matter of fact the only difference between sinus bradycardia rhythm and normal sinus rhythm is the heart rate. Because of this one variable, however, this sinus bradycardia rhythm is *not* normal.

    Sinus bradycardia is often called Sinus Brady. Recall from your knowledge of medical terminology, that the term "brady" means slow. In this rhythm, the SA node discharges impulses at a rate of less than 60 beats per minute.

    Sinus bradycardia may be caused by intrinsic disease of the SA node, vomiting, hypoxia, hypothermia, or the effects of certain drugs such as morphine, digitalis, verampamil, and some sedatives. Do we panic when we note a sinus bradycardia on a rhythm strip? No, we don't panic over *any* rhythm. We simply consider the ramifications of that rhythm, based on our patient's clinical condition. As a matter of fact, in a person who is sleeping and in a young, well-conditioned athlete, we expect to see some degree of sinus bradycardia as a normal phenomenon. Later in this chapter, we will discuss the clinical significance of this rhythm and other sinus dysrhythmias.

    Now, let's apply our five-step approach to analyzing this rhythm (Table 7–4 and Figure 7–2).

    Remember that sinus bradycardia looks very much like normal sinus rhythm, but the rate is slower (less than 60 beats per minute). **Remember, always monitor your patient's clinical condition.**

sinus bradycardia in this rhythm, the SA node discharges impulses at a rate of less than 60 beats per minute

SINUS TACHYCARDIA RHYTHM

This is the other "first cousin" of NSR. Tachycardia technically means a fast heart rate, and the term "sinus" tells us that this rhythm originated in the SA node. Thus we can conclude that **sinus tachycardia** is a variant of normal sinus rhythm, the only difference

sinus tachycardia a variant of normal sinus rhythm; the rate is generally considered to be 100–160 beats per minute

Table 7–4

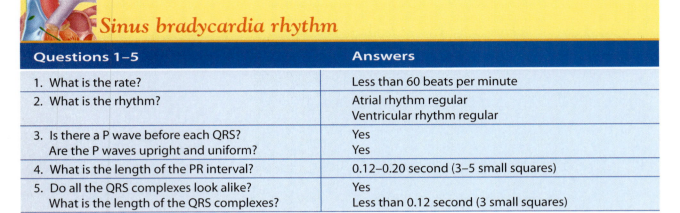

Questions 1–5	Answers
1. What is the rate?	Less than 60 beats per minute
2. What is the rhythm?	Atrial rhythm regular Ventricular rhythm regular
3. Is there a P wave before each QRS? Are the P waves upright and uniform?	Yes Yes
4. What is the length of the PR interval?	0.12–0.20 second (3–5 small squares)
5. Do all the QRS complexes look alike? What is the length of the QRS complexes?	Yes Less than 0.12 second (3 small squares)

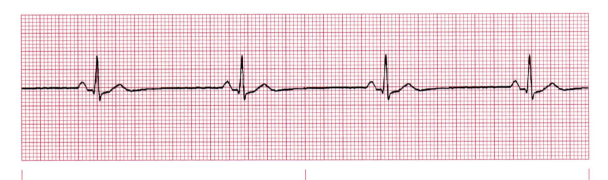

Figure 7–2. Sinus bradycardia rhythm

being the rate of the impulses generated by the SA node. The rate of sinus tachycardia, or sinus tach, is generally considered to be 100–160 beats per minute.

The impulses generated in this rhythm follow the normal pathway of the electrical conduction system. Thus P waves will be present before QRS complexes, the PR interval will be within normal limits, and the QRS complexes will all look similar and will be less than 0.12 second in length. The atrial and ventricular rhythms will be regular. As the heart rate approaches the upper limits of the normal range, the P waves may be slightly harder to discern, but they can usually be observed and analyzed.

Causes of sinus tachycardia are numerous, including exercise, fear, stress, anxiety, and ingestion of stimulants such as coffee or alcohol, all of which result in stimulation of the sympathetic nervous system. In addition, sinus tachycardia may result from hypovolemia, congestive heart failure, severe dehydration, or acute myocardial infarction. While it is generally held that sinus tachycardia, in and of itself, is not dangerous to the patient, we should remember that the underlying cause of this rhythm may be quite serious. If the very fast rate decreases the ability of the heart to refill properly, the patient's cardiac output may be reduced. In this instance it becomes very important that the underlying cause of the rhythm be identified and corrected as soon as possible. Remember that the KEY to properly identifying this rhythm is the **heart rate.**

Again, we will apply our five-step approach to analyzing this rhythm (Table 7–5 and Figure 7–3).

Remember that sinus tachycardia looks very much like normal sinus rhythm, but the rate is faster (more than 100 beats per minute). **Remember, always monitor your patient's clinical condition.**

Table 7–5

Sinus tachycardia rhythm

Questions 1–5	Answers
1. What is the rate?	100–160 bpm
2. What is the rhythm?	Atrial rhythm regular Ventricular rhythm regular
3. Is there a P wave before each QRS? Are the P waves upright and uniform?	Yes Yes
4. What is the length of the PR interval?	0.12–0.20 second (3–5 small squares)
5. Do all the QRS complexes look alike? What is the length of the QRS complexes?	Yes Less than 0.12 second (3 small squares)

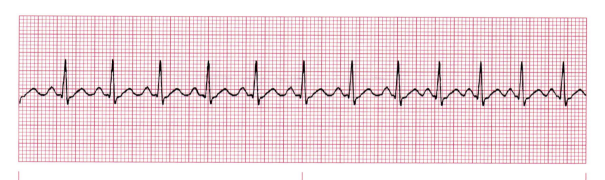

Figure 7–3.   Sinus tachycardia rhythm

SINUS DYSRHYTHMIA

Sinus dysrhythmia resembles other sinus rhythms, except for the slight irregularity of the heart rhythm. This rhythm is sometimes referred to as sinus arrhythmia. The rate of impulse formation in the SA node may vary with respirations. In this rhythm, impulses are initiated by the SA node, but at irregular intervals. An irregular rhythm is produced when the P-to-P intervals and the R-to-R intervals change with respirations. The heart rate increases during inspiration and decreases during expiration. As a general rule, there should be a difference of at least 0.08 second between the shortest and longest R-R intervals in order to determine that the rhythm is not a normal sinus rhythm. A very careful step-by-step approach is necessary to distinguish sinus dysrhythmia.

Sinus dysrhythmia is a common and normal finding, especially in children and young adults. Causes of sinus dysrhythmia may include the administration of certain drugs such as digitalis, underlying cardiac disease such as sick sinus syndrome, or myocardial infarction. Remember that the KEY to identifying this rhythm properly is the **heart rhythm.** Again, we will apply our five-step approach to analyzing this rhythm (Table 7–6 and Figure 7–4).

Remember that sinus dysrhythmia looks very much like normal sinus rhythm, but the rhythm is slightly irregular, varying with respirations. **Remember, always monitor your patient's clinical condition.**

sinus dysrhythmia an irregular rhythm produced when the P-to-P intervals and the R-to-R intervals change with respirations

Table 7–6

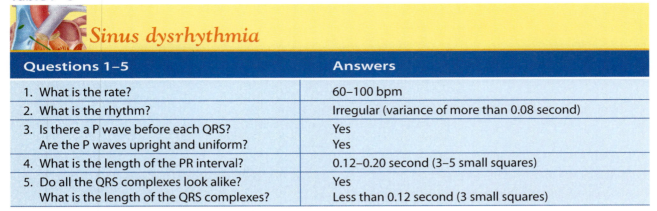

Sinus dysrhythmia	
Questions 1–5	**Answers**
1. What is the rate?	60–100 bpm
2. What is the rhythm?	Irregular (variance of more than 0.08 second)
3. Is there a P wave before each QRS?	Yes
Are the P waves upright and uniform?	Yes
4. What is the length of the PR interval?	0.12–0.20 second (3–5 small squares)
5. Do all the QRS complexes look alike?	Yes
What is the length of the QRS complexes?	Less than 0.12 second (3 small squares)

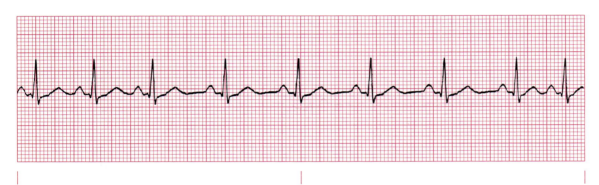

Figure 7–4. Sinus dysrhythmia rhythm

sinus arrest rhythm When the sinus node fails to discharge, the absence of a PQRST interval is noted on the rhythm strip

SINUS ARREST RHYTHM

When the SA node fails to initiate an impulse, a rhythm known as **sinus arrest** will result. When the sinus node fails to discharge, the absence of a PQRST interval is noted on the rhythm strip. This occurrence causes a slight period of cardiac standstill, which lasts until the sinus node continues its normal function. The absence of a PQRST complex appears as a pause on the EKG strip. This rhythm can quickly get your attention! However, if these occurrences are infrequent, there may be no immediate cause for undue concern. Patient assessment is imperative.

Causes of sinus arrest may include hypoxia, ischemia, damage to the SA node, or certain drugs such as digitalis or salicylates. Sinus arrest can also occur as a result of myocardial infarction. Remember that the KEY to properly identifying this rhythm is the **transient absence of the PQRST complexes.** Now, let's apply our five-step approach to analyzing this rhythm (Table 7–7 and Figure 7–5).

Remember that sinus arrest presents as an infrequent absence of a PQRST complex. **Remember, always monitor your patient's clinical condition.**

CLINICAL SIGNIFICANCE OF SINUS RHYTHMS

The clinical significance of sinus rhythms is directly associated with the assessment of your patient. Often, sinus rhythms are not particularly significant or serious. As with all rhythms, patient assessment is crucial to determining the patient's tolerance of the dys-

Table 7–7

Sinus arrest rhythm	
Questions 1–5	**Answers**
1. What is the rate?	Variable, depending on the frequency of sinus arrest
2. What is the rhythm?	Irregular, when sinus arrest is present
3. Is there a P wave before each QRS? Are the P waves upright and uniform?	Yes—if QRS is present Yes—if QRS is present
4. What is the length of the PR interval?	0.12–0.20 second (3–5 small squares)
5. Do all the QRS complexes look alike? What is the length of the QRS complexes?	Yes, when present Less than 0.12 second (3 small squares)

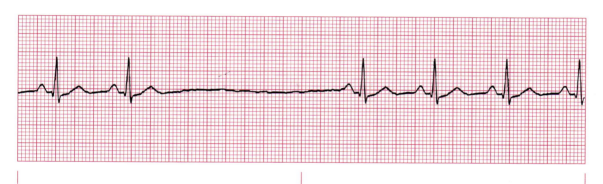

Figure 7–5.   Sinus arrest rhythm

rhythmia. Determine whether your patient is medically stable or medically unstable. If the patient is experiencing chest pains, dizziness, weakness, fainting, markedly de-creased or increased blood pressure, or alterations in level of consciousness, he or she is considered symptomatic or medically unstable. We will now discuss the clinical sig-nificance of each of the sinus dysrhythmias.

Sinus bradycardia

Recall now that sinus bradycardia is a dysrhythmia commonly seen in young, well-conditioned athletes or in people who are sleeping. However, if the patient's heart rate falls significantly, cardiac compromise will become a cause for concern. If your pa-tient becomes symptomatic, exhibiting signs of decreased cardiac output, treatment should be initiated at once. Treatment for sinus bradycardia may include the adminis-tration of oxygen, initiating an IV access line, administration of the drug Atropine, tran-scutaneous pacing (TCP), or some combination of these.

Signs of cardiac compromise may include, but are not limited to, the following: al-tered mental status, chest pain, hypotension, dizziness, and fainting. Be aware that si-nus bradycardia may follow the application of carotid sinus massage (discussed in Chapter 8). When the heart rate becomes extremely slow, ectopic (out-of-place) com-plexes or rhythms (like PVCs) may occur. Again, look at your patient and evaluate him or her continually.

Sinus tachycardia

Sinus tachycardia usually does not require treatment. Let me be quick to add, however, that it is imperative to seek out and correct the underlying cause of the rapid heart rate. In some cases, sinus tachycardia can be thought of as a double-edged sword. Why is this true? Because while sinus tachycardia may actually be a compensatory mechanism for decreased stroke volume, it is also true that cardiac output may fall when the heart rate approaches 150 bpm, due to inadequate ventricular filling time. In addition, myocardial oxygen demand increases with rapid heart rates, and this can precipitate myocardial ischemia or even infarct of the myocardial tissue. It should also be noted that sinus tachycardia may result from the administration of drugs such as epinephrine or from certain stimulants, such as cocaine or excessive amounts of caffeine.

Treatment of sinus tachycardia is aimed at finding and treating the underlying cause. If the patient is hypovolemic, the hypovolemia should be corrected as soon as is feasible. If the patient is complaining of chest pain, oxygen should be administered immediately and the patient should be moved to a definitive care facility. Often, when the underlying cause of this dysrhythmia is identified and managed, the rhythm will gradually convert back to the patient's normal rhythm.

Sinus dysrhythmia

Sinus dysrhythmia is considered a normal alteration in heart rhythm, especially in young children and elderly adults people. This rhythm usually does not require emergency intercession.

Sinus arrest

By now, I'm quite sure you have absorbed the idea that all patients, even those with "normal" heart rhythms, must be constantly monitored and assessed. As I mentioned earlier in this chapter, sinus arrest rhythm usually demands our immediate attention, just by virtue of its appearance on the oscilloscope or rhythm strip.

When you begin to analyze a rhythm strip that shows sinus arrest, you (of course) ask the first question: "What is the patient's heart rate?" As soon as you begin to calculate heart rate, you immediately notice that *something* (namely, a PQRST complex) is missing! Right away, you know that something is wrong, so you look at your patient (yes, again). If the patient appears to be medically stable, you continue with your analysis of the strip.

If your patient is asymptomatic (medically stable) and the episodes of sinus arrest are occurring only occasionally, continued observation may be all that is required. It is prudent to keep in mind that frequent episodes of sinus arrest may cause cardiac compromise. If the patient is bradycardic and exhibits other accompanying symptoms (feelings of faintness or dizziness), it may be necessary to administer the drug called atropine. If atropine is ineffective, transcutaneous pacing (TCP) may be indicated.

SUMMARY

Rhythms that arise from the SA node include normal sinus rhythm, sinus bradycardia, sinus tachycardia, sinus dysrhythmia, and sinus arrest. Common characteristics of the sinus rhythms include the usually normal appearance of P wave morphology, upright P waves in Lead II, and the normal duration of the PR interval and the QRS complex. The only "normal" rhythm is normal sinus rhythm; all other rhythms in this group are appropriately termed *dysrhythmias*.

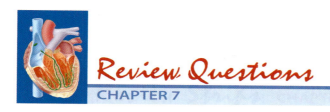

Review Questions
CHAPTER 7

1. How many chambers are located in the heart?
   a. Five
   b. Three
   c. Four
   d. Six

2. The two upper chambers of the heart are called the:
   a. Ventricles
   b. Atria
   c. Aorta
   d. Vena cava

3. What happens to the blood as it passes through the pulmonary capillaries?
   a. Oxygen is added and carbon dioxide removed.
   b. Carbon dioxide is added and oxygen is removed.
   c. Oxygen is added and carbon dioxide is added.
   d. Oxygen is removed and carbon dioxide is removed.

4. The right ventricle pumps oxygen-poor blood to the lungs through the:
   a. Pulmonary veins
   b. Aorta
   c. Vena cava
   d. Pulmonary arteries

5. What is the normal order of the electrical conduction pattern of the heart?
   a. AV node, SA node, ventricles
   b. Ventricles, AV node, SA node
   c. SA node, ventricles, AV node
   d. SA node, AV node, ventricles

6. An abnormal rhythm of the heart is called a:
   a. Dysrhythmia
   b. Paranormal rhythm
   c. Rhythmia
   d. Pararhythm

PACs sometimes occur in patterns such as pairs (two sequential PACs), atrial bigeminy (every other beat is a PAC), or atrial trigeminy (every third beat is a PAC). When you are counting the rate of a rhythm containing a PAC, it is important to remember that you should note the entire count of R waves of the PAC.

Premature atrial complexes may be caused by many different events. Causes of PACs may include the use of stimulants (caffeine, alcohol), hypoxia, increased sympathetic tone, imbalances of electrolytes, digitalis toxicity, or underlying cardiovascular disease. In some cases, isolated PACs may occur without cause.

Because this discussion is our first mention of **premature** beats or complexes, this is an appropriate time for you to recognize a very important fact—when any premature beat occurs more than six times per minute, the dysrhythmia assumes more importance and is called "frequent." For instance, the rhythm may be called sinus bradycardia with frequent PACs. An increase in the frequency of premature beats indicates significant irritability of myocardial tissues and becomes a definite cause for concern. Be aware that more serious dysrhythmias may develop in the presence of frequent premature beats.

Now that we've examined the prominent characteristics of a premature atrial complex, let's explore the five-step approach to interpreting this rhythm. We'll ask the five questions that will enable us to identify the rhythm definitively and correctly. (See Table 8–2 and Figure 8–3.)

Table 8–2

Premature atrial complexes

Questions 1–5	Answers
1. What is the rate?	Usually normal
2. What is the rhythm?	Usually regular, except for PAC
3. Is there a P wave before each QRS? Are the P waves upright and uniform?	Differs in shape, size, and location from normal P waves of rhythm
4. What is the length of the PR interval?	Variable, depending on pacemaker site
5. Do all the QRS complexes look alike? What is the length of the QRS complexes?	Similar to QRS of underlying rhythm; usually less than 0.12 second (3 small squares)

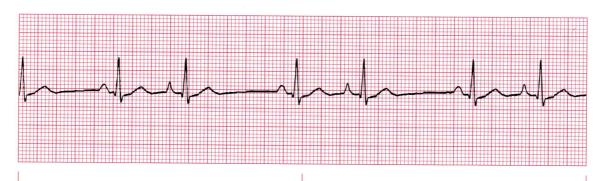

Figure 8–3.   Premature atrial complexes

Remember that the PAC often appears as an "ectopic" (or out-of-place) beat in an otherwise regular rhythm. **Remember: always monitor your patient's clinical condition!**

REENTRY DYSRHYTHMIAS

Reentry can be defined as the reactivation of myocardial tissue for a second or subsequent time by the same electrical impulse. Although reentry is a common dysrhythmic mechanism, it is a complicated event. This concept can be thought of as a "short circuit" of the heart's electrical conduction system.

Reentry develops when the course of an electrical impulse is delayed or blocked in one or more segments of the heart's electrical conduction system. Because of this delay, the electrical impulse is allowed to travel in only one direction (unilateral). As the impulse moves in a cycle throughout the heart tissue, a series of fast depolarization ensues (Figure 8–4).

Causes of reentry due to conduction delays or blocks include hyperkalemia, myocardial ischemia, and certain antidysrhythmic medications. Specific rhythms associated with reentry include atrial flutter, atrial fibrillation, paroxysmal supraventricular tachycardia, and premature atrial complexes.

reentry the reactivation of myocardial tissue for a second or subsequent time by the same electrical impulse

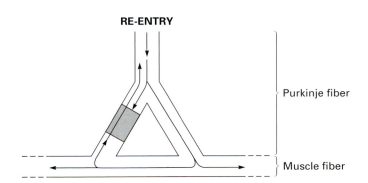

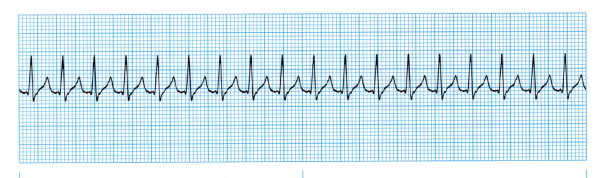

Figure 8–4.   Reentry is a phenomenon usually created by a one-way block that causes a wave of depolarization to be rapidly propagated in a circular motion. Upper: Schematic drawing. Lower: EKG tracing.

ATRIAL FLUTTER RHYTHM

Another common atrial dysrhythmia is called atrial flutter. Atrial flutter is characterized by the presence of regular atrial activity with a picket-fence or sawtooth pattern. Think **sawtooth!** This rhythm is often a favorite of students who are initially learning EKG interpretation because it is generally easy to recognize.

atrial flutter
when a single irritable site in the atria initiates many electrical impulses at a rapid rate, characterized by the presence of regular atrial activity with a picket-fence or **sawtooth** pattern

When a single irritable site in the atria initiates many electrical impulses at a rapid rate, the rhythm is called **atrial flutter.** Normal P waves are not produced in atrial flutter, because electrical impulses are conducted throughout the atria at a very rapid rate. Rather than the presence of normally appearing P waves, flutter (or sawtooth) waves, also known as F waves, are patterned.

The AV node plays a very important role in atrial flutter rhythms: it truly becomes the "gatekeeper" to the ventricles. The ventricular response rate is based on the number of impulses that the AV node accepts. In other words, if every other flutter impulse is blocked by the AV node, the conduction ratio becomes 2 to 1—there will be two atrial contractions for each ventricular contraction. If the AV node conducts only one of every four atrial contractions, the conduction ratio is 4 to 1; thus, an atrial rate of 300 bpm will parallel a ventricular rate of 75 bpm. If the conduction ratio changes or varies frequently, an irregular ventricular rate will result. In addition, if the conduction ratio is 2 to 1, the F waves may be more difficult to recognize. Atrial flutter with a ventricular rate of less than 60 bpm is atrial flutter with a **slow ventricular response**. A ventricular rate of 100–150 bpm is atrial flutter with a **rapid ventricular response**.

slow ventricular response a ventricular rate of less than 60 bpm

rapid ventricular response a ventricular rate of 100–150 bpm

Causes of atrial flutter include acute myocardial infarction, hypoxia, digitalis toxicity, congestive heart failure, SA node disease, and pulmonary embolism. Atrial flutter may occur in patients with normal, healthy hearts, but it is most often seen in elderly patients with underlying chronic heart disease.

We will now examine the five-step approach to interpreting this rhythm. As always, you must ask the five basic questions that will permit you to identify this rhythm conclusively. (See Table 8–3 and Figure 8–5.)

Recall that the **key** to interpreting atrial flutter is the presence of a **sawtooth pattern. Remember: always monitor your patient's clinical condition!**

Table 8–3

Atrial flutter

Questions 1–5	Answers
1. What is the rate?	Atrial: 250–300 bpm Ventricular: variable
2. What is the rhythm?	Atrial: regular; Ventricular: regular or irregular
3. Is there a P wave before each QRS? Are the P waves upright and uniform?	Normal P waves are absent; replaced by F waves (sawtooth)
4. What is the length of the PR interval?	Not measurable
5. Do all the QRS complexes look alike? What is the length of the QRS complexes?	Usually less than 0.12 second (3 small squares)

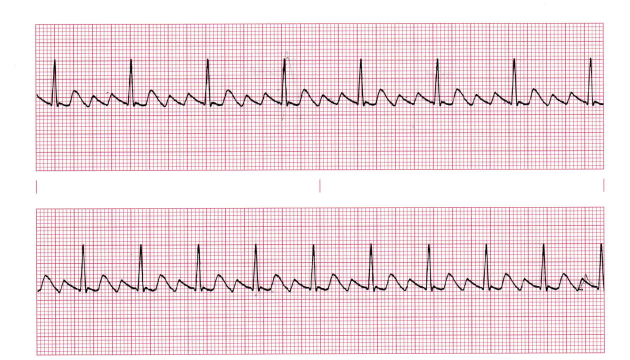

Figure 8–5.   Atrial flutter

ATRIAL FIBRILLATION RHYTHM

Atrial fibrillation is one of the most common atrial dysrhythmias encountered in elderly patients. Typically, atrial fibrillation presents with three definite characteristics. First, there is a notable absence of P waves in this rhythm. Second, P waves are replaced by *f* waves, or fibrillatory waves. Third, possibly the most obvious characteristic of atrial fibrillation is that the ventricular response rate is totally irregular—it is called an *irregular irregularity.* The QRS complexes in an atrial fibrillation rhythm are usually within normal limits.

When multiple disorganized ectopic atrial foci generate electrical activity at a very rapid rate (atrial rate varies from 350 to 750 bpm), **atrial fibrillation** results. The ventricular response rate is 140–200 bpm in the **untreated** atrial fibrillation rhythms. In this rhythm, multiple ectopic foci from within the atria are literally blitzing the AV node. It is pathophysiologically impossible for the AV node to handle or conduct each of these impulses. Consequently, the AV node allows impulses to enter the conduction system pathway completely at random. This random selection of impulse passage through the AV node accounts for the total irregularity of the rhythm called atrial fibrillation. In the truest sense of EKG interpretation, atrial fibrillation is an irregular irregularity in heart rhythm.

Frequently, we find ourselves shortening or abbreviating the pronunciation of this rhythm; however, I discourage my students from this practice because the abbreviated terms "a-fib" and "v-fib" sound very much alike but indicate *very different* rhythms. It's easier to be safe and take another millisecond to pronounce both words—atrial fibrillation!

As we address the causes of atrial fibrillation, it is important to note that this rhythm may be chronic in nature and is quite commonly associated with underlying heart disease such as congestive heart failure or rheumatic heart disease. This rhythm may also be associated with acute myocardial infarction, hypoxia, myocardial ischemia, or digitalis toxicity.

atrial fibrillation
when multiple disorganized ectopic atrial foci generate electrical activity at a very rapid rate (atrial rate varies from 350 to 750 bpm)

The goal of therapy when treating atrial fibrillation with a rapid ventricular response is to slow the ventricular response to somewhere within a range of 80–100 bpm. This can sometimes be accomplished with the careful, monitored administration of digitalis.

While considering this rhythm, one might visualize the atria as though they are "quivering." When this occurs, the atria do not contract productively. Thus the effectiveness of myocardial contraction is decreased because the atria are not forcefully filling the ventricles with blood. As with the majority of dysrhythmias, a new occurrence of atrial fibrillation is usually treated when discovered, as it can indicate an increase in irritability within the atrial tissue.

Recall now that irritability in myocardial tissue can signal progression to a more serious dysrhythmia. Ask yourself how well your patient is tolerating this rhythm. If your patient is clinically symptomatic and you elect to administer oxygen, do the symptoms abate after the oxygen is administered? If not, you must then consider what course of action to follow.

As we examine the five step approach to interpreting this rhythm, contemplate your concerns about the clinical condition of an imagined patient and decisively identify this rhythm. Again, do not be shy or hesitant about asking for guidance if you falter during the initial trial of rhythm interpretation. Remember, there are no stupid questions. There are just questions that are unasked and thus unanswered. **Hint: Think "irregular irregularity"**—it just may be atrial fibrillation. (See Table 8–4 and Figure 8–6.)

Table 8–4

Atrial fibrillation

Questions 1–5	Answers
1. What is the rate?	Atrial: 350–400 bpm Ventricular: variable
2. What is the rhythm?	Irregularly irregular
3. Is there a P wave before each QRS? Are the P waves upright and uniform?	Normal P waves are absent; replaced by f waves
4. What is the length of the PR interval?	Not discernable
5. Do all the QRS complexes look alike? What is the length of the QRS complexes?	Yes Usually less than 0.10 second

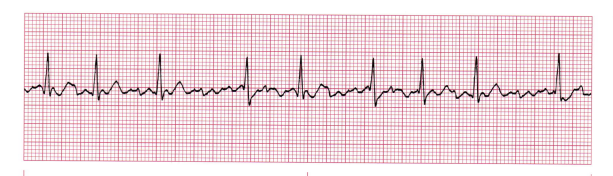

Figure 8–6.   Atrial fibrillation

Recall that the **key** to interpreting atrial fibrillation is the **presence of an irregularly irregular pattern and an absence of P waves. Remember: Always monitor your patient's clinical condition!**

SUPRAVENTRICULAR TACHYCARDIA RHYTHMS

Supraventricular tachycardia (SVT) is a general term that encompasses all fast (tachy-) dysrhythmias in which the heart rate is greater than 100 bpm. Technically, even sinus tachycardia is a supraventricular tachycardia, in that it is a rhythm arising above (supra) the ventricles (ventricular). Generally, we think of SVT as the "big umbrella" title of dysrhythmias, under which cascades a host of specific rhythms: paroxysmal supraventricular tachycardia (PSVT), paroxysmal atrial tachycardia (PAT), atrial tachycardia (AT), paroxysmal junctional tachycardia (PJT), multifocal atrial tachycardia (MAT), and junctional tachycardia (JT). Thus the term "supraventricular tachycardia" technically applies to any tachycardia rhythm originating above the ventricle.

It is wise to attempt to identify where the rhythm is originating in order to get a good idea of which type of SVT you are observing. Differential diagnosis of the exact type of SVT being observed is not critical in the emergent situation and should never delay patient care. Look at your patient. **Treat the patient, not the monitor!**

The term **"paroxysmal"** refers to a sudden onset or cessation or both. In order to label a rhythm correctly as paroxysmal, it is critical that the sudden onset or cessation be observed on the cardiac monitor. Only then, in the strictest sense, can the rhythm be **correctly** identified as paroxysmal in nature. Typically, bouts of PSVT begin and end abruptly. Notably, these bouts may continue for several hours or for only a few seconds.

Supraventricular tachycardia occurs when a rapid atrial ectopic focus overrides the SA node and become the heart's primary pacemaker. Supraventricular tachycardia can resemble a rapid sinus tachycardia; thus careful calculation of the heart rate is important. Recall that sinus tachycardia seldom exceeds 160–170 bpm at the high-rate range. In both these dysrhythmias, the QRS complexes are typically normal in appearance. When P waves are present, they have a consistent relationship with the QRS complexes. In SVT rhythms, P waves are often hidden in the T waves of the preceding complex and thus may be difficult, if not impossible, to discern.

Causes of the SVT rhythms are similar, in part, to the causes of other atrial dysrhythmias. Although SVT is not a common finding in the setting of an acute myocardial infarction, this rhythm may be associated with underlying cardiovascular diseases such as rheumatic heart disease and atherosclerotic cardiovascular disease. Supraventricular tachycardia may occur in a healthy person and can result from overexertion, stress, hypoxia, excessive use of stimulants, or hypokalemia.

Methods utilized to stimulate baroreceptors (located in the internal carotid and aortic arch) are called **vagal maneuvers.** When these receptors are stimulated, the vagus nerve releases acetylcholine, resulting in slowing of the heart rate. Examples of vagal maneuvers include asking the patient to bear down (as in an attempt to move the bowels), cough, or squat, and using carotid sinus massage. (Carotid sinus massage must be avoided with older patients and only performed unilaterally.)

Let's examine the five-step approach to interpreting this rhythm. **Hint:** Think, **"What is the heart rate, and can I see definite P waves?"** (See Table 8–5 and Figure 8–7.)

supraventricular tachycardia (SVT) a general term that encompasses all fast (tachy-) dysrhythmias in which the heart rate is greater than 100 bpm

paroxysmal refers to a sudden onset or cessation or both

vagal maneuvers methods utilized to stimulate baroreceptors (located in the internal carotid and aortic arch); when these receptors are stimulated, the vagus nerve releases acetylcholine, resulting in slowing of the heart rate

Table 8–5

Supraventricular tachycardia

Questions 1–5	Answers
1. What is the rate?	Atrial: 150–250 bpm Ventricular: 150–250 bpm
2. What is the rhythm?	Regular
3. Is there a P wave before each QRS? Are the P waves upright and uniform?	Usually not discernible, especially at the high-rate range
4. What is the length of the PR interval?	Usually not discernible
5. Do all the QRS complexes look alike? What is the length of the QRS complexes?	Yes Usually less than 0.10 second

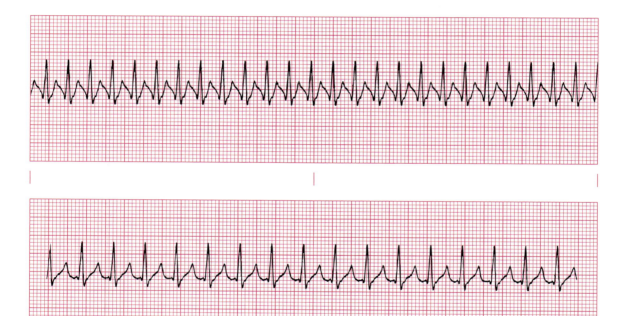

Figure 8–7. Supraventricular tachycardia

Remember that the patient who is experiencing PSVT may complain of a feeling that his or her heart is "running away" or "racing." **Remember: it is critical to determine whether the patient is symptomatic or nonsymptomatic; therefore, always monitor your patient's clinical condition!**

WOLFF-PARKINSON-WHITE (WPW) SYNDROME

In the late 1800s, an American physician, Louis Wolff; an English cardiologist, Sir John Parkinson; and an American cardiologist, Paul Dudley White, identified the preexcita-

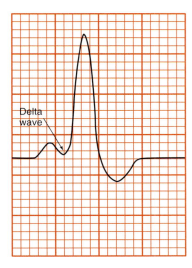

Figure 8–8.   Delta wave of Wolff-Parkinson-White syndrome

tion syndrome called **Wolff-Parkinson-White syndrome,** or **WPW.** This atrioventricular conduction disorder is characterized by two AV conduction pathways and is often identified by a characteristic delta wave seen on an electrocardiogram at the beginning of the QRS complex.

In WPW syndrome, the QRS complex is greater than 0.10 second, because the ventricles are stimulated by an impulse that originated outside the normal conduction pathway. Wolff-Parkinson-White syndrome is thought to be congenital. If P waves are identifiable in WPW rhythms, the PR interval may be 0.12 second or longer because the AV node is bypassed. This disorder is associated with a high incidence of tachydysrhythmias. Treatment of WPW, if required, is based on the underlying rhythm as well as the patient's clinical condition (Figure 8–8).

CLINICAL SIGNIFICANCE OF ATRIAL RHYTHMS

Wandering atrial pacemaker rhythm

Wandering atrial pacemaker rhythms are not typically clinically significant. The patient is usually asymptomatic, but it should be noted that WAP can be a precursor of other atrial dysrhythmias. This rhythm may be caused by digitalis toxicity; therefore, the patient's digitalis blood level must be closely monitored, and the medication should be adjusted accordingly.

Premature atrial contraction (complex)

In a person with a healthy heart, isolated PACs are not significant. As with many other dysrhythmias, PACs may be corrected by identifying and treating the underlying cause.

Frequent PACs (more than 6 per minute) may signify underlying heart disease and may initiate other atrial dysrhythmias, such as atrial fibrillation, atrial tachycardia, PSVT, or atrial flutter.

Wolff-Parkinson-White syndrome, (WPW)
preexcitation syndrome and atrioventricular conduction disorder characterized by two AV conduction pathways and is often identified by a characteristic delta wave seen on an electrocardiogram at the beginning of the QRS complex

Atrial flutter rhythm

The clinical significance of atrial flutter is directly related to the patient's clinical condition. If the ventricular rate is normal, the rhythm is generally well tolerated. If the ventricular response rate is fast, a decrease in cardiac output may occur, resulting in symptoms. As ventricular response rates increase, the patient may complain of dizziness, weakness, chest pain, or palpitations. In cases of rapid ventricular response rates, treatment may be directed toward decreasing the ventricular rate with medication. If the patient's symptoms progress and the patient becomes hemodynamically unstable, cardioversion may be indicated.

The initial setting for synchronized cardioversion is 50–100 joules in atrial flutter rhythms. Recall also that oxygen therapy is the first and most important therapy for patients who are exhibiting signs or symptoms of compromised cardiac output, regardless of the cause.

Atrial fibrillation rhythm

If the patient does not exhibit signs or symptoms, no treatment may be required. This is often the case in patients with controlled atrial fibrillation. Cardiac output can fall, due to ventricular response rates of less than 60. In cases of rapid ventricular response rates, treatment may be directed toward decreasing the ventricular rate with the administration of medications. If the patient's symptoms progress and the patient becomes hemodynamically unstable, cardioversion may be indicated and should be initiated at 50–100 joules, depending on the physician's preference.

It is wise to keep in mind that the atria do not empty sufficiently in rapid atrial fibrillation rhythms. Lack of atrial activity causes a 30% decrease in cardiac output. Because the **"atrial kick"** (the final phase of diastole) is lost, blood tends to stagnate in the atria. These patients are at risk for the development of atrial and systemic emboli and must be carefully monitored.

atrial kick the final phase of diastole, atrial contraction forces remaining blood into the ventricles: provides 15–30% of ventricular filling

Supraventricular tachycardia rhythms

Supraventricular rhythms may occur in a patient with a healthy heart and may be well tolerated for short intervals. The patient may complain the heart is "racing" or "running away" (a common description of palpitations) and may appear very anxious or excited. If the patient is symptomatic, treatment is directed at slowing the heart rate by the use of vagal maneuvers, drug therapy, or synchronized cardioversion (initial setting of 100 joules).

Prolonged episodes of SVT may increase myocardial oxygen demand and may thus increase the need for supplemental oxygen therapy. Always administer oxygen to patients who are exhibiting any signs or symptoms of cardiac compromise. To determine the appropriate course of treatment, you must observe and assess your patient's clinical condition.

SUMMARY

Dysrhythmias that originate in the atrial tissues, or in the internodal pathways, are referred to as atrial dysrhythmias. Atrial dysrhythmias arise from many causes, including hypoxia, ischemia, and atrial enlargement secondary to congestive heart failure. As with the treatment and management of all patients exhibiting dysrhythmias, excellent patient assessment skills are critically important.

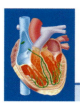

Review Questions
CHAPTER 8

1. Vagal maneuvers are performed to:
   a. Slow the heart rate
   b. Dilate the coronary arteries
   c. Reduce ventricular irritability
   d. Improve conduction through the AV node

2. The coronary arteries receive oxygenated blood from the:
   a. Aorta
   b. Coronary sinus
   c. Pulmonary veins
   d. Pulmonary arteries

3. When any premature beat occurs more than six times per minute, the dysrhythmia assumes more importance and is called:
   a. Regular
   b. Frequent
   c. Irregular
   d. Continual

4. The initial setting for cardioversion is _____ joules in atrial flutter rhythms.
   a. 200–250
   b. 150–200
   c. 200–300
   d. 50–100

5. The electrocardiogram is used to:
   a. Determine pulse rate
   b. Detect valvular dysfunction
   c. Evaluate electrical activity in the heart
   d. Determine whether the heart is beating

6. Most atrial fibrillation waves are not followed by a QRS complex because the:
   a. Impulses are initiated in the left ventricle
   b. Stimuli are not strong enough to be conducted
   c. Ventricle can receive only 120 stimuli in one minute
   d. AV junction is unable to conduct all the excitation impulses

7. "Supraventricular rhythm" means that the impulse, or stimulus, arises above the ventricles.

   a. True

   b. False

8. PAT is a sudden onset of atrial tachycardia.

   a. True

   b. False

9. The T wave on the EKG strip represents:

   a. Rest period

   b. Bundle of His

   c. Atrial contraction

   d. Ventricular contraction

10. When interpreting dysrhythmias, you must remember that the most important key is the:

    a. PR interval

    b. Rate and rhythm

    c. Presence of dysrhythmias

    d. Patient's clinical appearance

11. Premature atrial complexes may occur in any rhythm but are much easier to identify in any bradycardic rhythm.

    a. True

    b. False

12. For a diagnosis of wandering atrial pacemaker, observation of at least _____ different P waves is required.

    a. Two

    b. Three

    c. Four

    d. Six

13. Methods used to stimulate baroreceptors (located in the internal carotid and aortic arch) are called _____ maneuvers.

    a. Reflex

    b. Vasal

    c. Vagal

    d. Sinus

14. When a single irritable site in the atria initiates many electrical impulses at a rapid rate, the rhythm is called:

    a. Sinus rhythm

    b. Atrial flutter

    c. Atrial fibrillation

    d. Atrial tachycardia

15. SVT may occur in a healthy person and can result from:

    a. Overexertion

    b. Hypoxia

    c. Hypokalemia

    d. All of the above

 Review Strips   CHAPTER 8

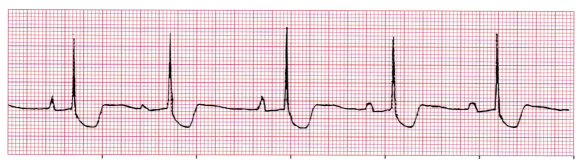

1. Rate _____ Rhythm _____

    P wave_____ PR interval_____

    QRS complex_____ Interpretation _____

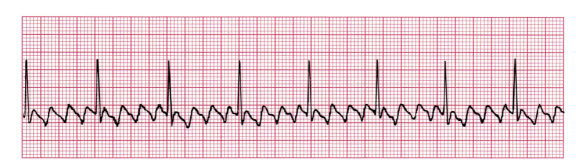

2. Rate _____ Rhythm _____

    P wave_____ PR interval_____

    QRS complex_____ Interpretation _____

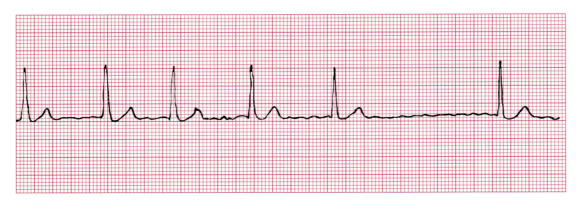

3. Rate _____ Rhythm _____

P wave _____ PR interval _____

QRS complex _____ Interpretation _____

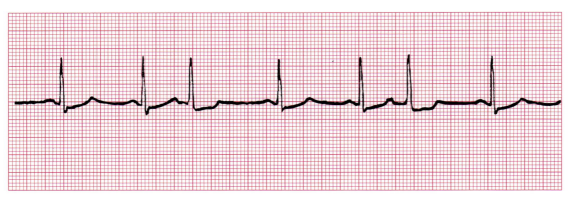

4. Rate _____ Rhythm _____

P wave _____ PR interval _____

QRS complex _____ Interpretation _____

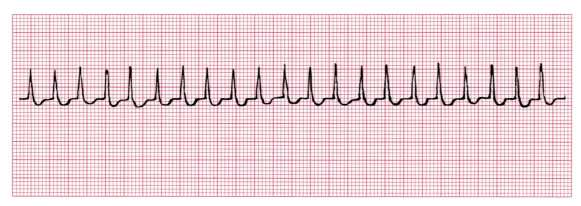

5. Rate _____ Rhythm _____

P wave _____ PR interval _____

QRS complex _____ Interpretation _____

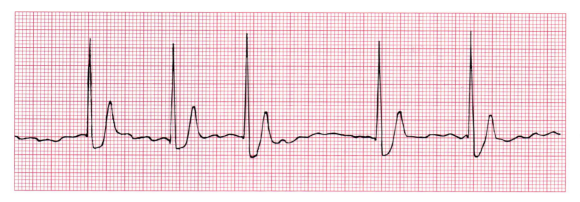

6. Rate _____   Rhythm _____
  P wave _____   PR interval _____
  QRS complex _____   Interpretation _____

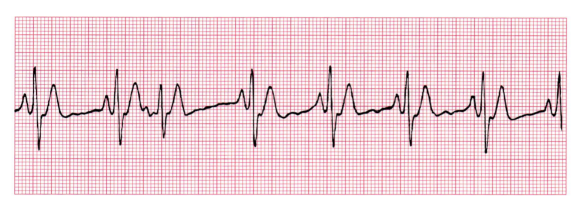

7. Rate _____   Rhythm _____
  P wave _____   PR interval _____
  QRS complex _____   Interpretation _____

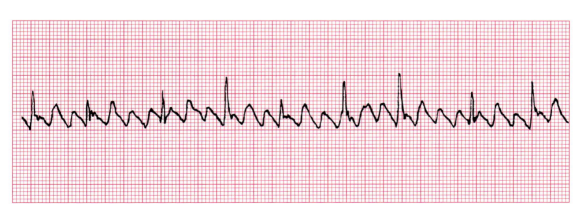

8. Rate _____   Rhythm _____
  P wave _____   PR interval _____
  QRS complex _____   Interpretation _____

INTRODUCTION

In Chapters 7 and 8, we discussed sinus rhythms and atrial rhythms. We learned that the SA node is the primary pacemaker in the heart and that impulses sometimes arise from the atria. For various reasons, such as drug toxicity or underlying cardiac disease, the SA node and the atria may fail to initiate electrical impulses. If this failure develops, the secondary pacemaker of the heart, the AV junction, will assume the role of pacing the heart.

It may be helpful for you to recognize that all junctional dysrhythmias contain several similar EKG features. These common features include P waves that are inverted or absent, a PR interval that is usually less than 0.12 second in duration, and QRS complexes that are within normal limits.

ORIGIN OF JUNCTIONAL RHYTHMS

junctional rhythms rhythms that are initiated in the area of the AV junction

Rhythms that are initiated in the area of the AV junction are called **junctional rhythms.** Formerly, rhythms originating in the AV node were called nodal rhythms. Technically, and in reference to pathophysiology of the heart, "junctional" is a more accurate term than "nodal." Thus in this chapter we will discuss the more common junctional rhythms. Although junctional rhythms are not considered lethal or life-threatening rhythms, you should recall that *patient assessment* is the most important indicator of the clinical significance of any dysrhythmia.

REVIEW OF THE ELECTRICAL CONDUCTION SYSTEM

We learned earlier in this text that the SA node is the heart's primary pacemaker. If the SA node fails to initiate impulses, the AV junction may assume the important role of pacing the heart. When the AV junction becomes the dominant pacemaker of the heart, the atria may or may not be stimulated. In order for the atria to be activated, the electrical impulses must travel in a retrograde (backward) direction from the AV junction. Therefore, the presence, absence, and location of P waves become key factors in the interpretation of junctional rhythms.

P WAVES

Recall now that we normally expect to see P waves *before* each QRS complex. However, because the electrical impulse in a junctional rhythm is traveling away from the positive electrode in Leads II and III, the P wave will be inverted or negative. At times, the P wave will not be seen, if atrial and ventricular depolarization occur simultaneously. In this case, the P wave is hidden in the QRS complex. At other times, the atria will depolarize after the ventricles have depolarized. When this occurs, an inverted P wave will appear *after* the QRS complex.

On the basis of this information, you should remember that a P wave may be seen before or after the QRS complex, or it may not be visible at all, in a junctional rhythm. You should recognize that the retrograde movement of the electrical impulses in junctional dysrhythmias accounts for all three of the distinctive changes in the P waves.

PREMATURE JUNCTIONAL CONTRACTIONS

Formerly called premature nodal contractions (PNCs), **premature junctional contractions (PJCs)** are initiated from a single site in the AV junction and arise earlier than the next anticipated complex of the underlying rhythm. If the SA node is depolarized by the ectopic beat, a noncompensatory pause occurs. Recall now that a **noncompensatory pause** (as we learned in our discussion of PACs in Chapter 8) is the pause that occurs after an ectopic beat, when the SA node is depolarized. Because of this noncompensatory pause, the underlying rhythm of the heart is interrupted. Premature junctional contractions can also result in a **compensatory pause** (a pause that occurs after an ectopic beat in which the SA node is unaffected and the cadence of the heart is uninterrupted). Therefore, we recognize that PJCs can result in either a compensatory or a noncompensatory pause, depending on whether the SA node is influenced by the ectopic beat.

Premature junctional contractions, or complexes, are less common than premature atrial complexes (PACs, discussed in Chapter 8) or premature ventricular contractions (PVCs, to be discussed in Chapter 10) and may occur in any rhythm. As with all ectopic beats, it is easier to identify PJCs when the rhythm is sinus or bradycardic. Also as with other premature beats, you should remember to determine the heart rate by counting the total number of R waves (including the R wave of the PJC). In addition, when interpreting a rhythm strip containing a PJC, you must determine the underlying rhythm. For example, a strip of sinus rhythm that includes one PJC would be called *sinus rhythm with a PJC*.

Causes of PJCs may include fever, anxiety, exercise, drug effects, stimulants, hypoxia, or myocardial ischemia. Premature junctional complexes may occur without any definite underlying cause. It is important to note that isolated occurrences of PJCs are not life-threatening. However, as with any dysrhythmia, the patient should be monitored closely because more serious dysrhythmias may be precipitated by ectopic foci.

Now it's time to apply the five-step approach to rhythm analysis in order to recognize a PJC correctly. Remember: When analyzing a static (stationary, paper) strip, **always** study the strip from left to right. (See Table 9–1 and Figure 9–1.)

premature junctional contractions (PJCs) initiate from a single site in the AV junction and arise earlier than the next anticipated complex of the underlying rhythm

noncompensatory pause the pause that occurs after an ectopic beat, when the SA node is depolarized

compensatory pause a pause that occurs after an ectopic beat in which the SA node is unaffected and the cadence of the heart is uninterrupted

Table 9–1

Premature junctional complexes

Questions 1–5	Answers
1. What is the rate?	Rate of underlying rhythm, plus the PJC or PJCs
2. What is the rhythm?	Usually regular, except for premature beat (PJC)
3. Is there a P wave before each QRS? Are the P waves upright and uniform?	Inverted or absent; may appear before or after the QRS
4. What is the length of the PR interval?	Usually less than 0.12 second if P wave precedes QRS; absent if no P wave occurs before the QRS
5. Do all the QRS complexes look alike? What is the length of the QRS complexes?	Yes Less than 0.12 second, if no defect in ventricular conduction

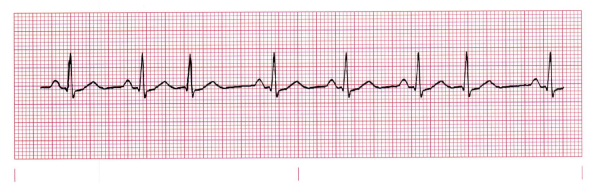

Figure 9–1.   Premature junctional complexes

Remember that the appearance of the P wave (inverted, absent, or occurring after the QRS) is the **key** to discerning the presence of premature junctional complexes. **Remember: Always monitor your patient's clinical condition!**

JUNCTIONAL ESCAPE RHYTHMS

If you recall our discussion of the electrical conduction system of the heart (Chapter 4), you will remember learning about the hearts' pacemakers. We know that the heart is indeed an amazing organ. If, for any of a number of reasons, the SA node fails to generate an impulse or if the rate of impulse generation falls below that of the AV node, then the AV node will assume the role of the pacemaker. When this occurs, the resulting rhythm is called a **junctional escape rhythm.** The ability of the AV node to assume this role is a safety feature of the heart. Recall now that the intrinsic rate of the AV node is 40–60 beats per minute (bpm).

If an isolated junctional beat occurs, it is called a *junctional escape beat (or complex).* If a series of junctional escape beats occur, the rhythm is then called a *junctional escape rhythm.* Remember that, as we discussed earlier in this chapter, the P wave may not be seen if atrial and ventricular depolarization occur simultaneously.

Causes of junctional escape beats or junctional escape rhythm include SA node disease, hypoxia, increased parasympathetic (vagal) tone, certain cardiac drugs, and a complete heart block. A patient with a junctional escape rhythm may be symptomatic or asymptomatic. If the patient is symptomatic, the treatment will be based on the underlying cause of the dysrhythmia.

The five-step approach should now be applied to the rhythm represented in Table 9–2 and Figure 9–2.

Remember that the rate of a junctional escape rhythm will be the intrinsic rate of the AV junctional tissue (40–60 bpm) and the P waves may be inverted or absent or may occur after the QRS complexes. **Remember: Always monitor your patient's clinical condition!**

ACCELERATED JUNCTIONAL RHYTHMS

In our earlier discussion of the properties of the heart, we addressed the term "automaticity." This term refers to the capability of the pacemaker cells of the heart to self-depolarize. Increased automaticity in the AV junction, causing the junction to discharge impulses at a rate faster than its intrinsic rate, results in a dysrhythmia referred to as **accelerated junctional rhythm.**

junctional escape rhythm when the SA node fails to generate an impulse or if the rate of impulse generation falls below that of the AV node, then the AV node will assume the role of the pacemaker, the resulting rhythm is called a junctional escape rhythm

accelerated junctional rhythm increased automaticity in the AV junction, causing the junction to discharge impulses at a rate faster than its intrinsic rate

Table 9–2

Junctional escape rhythm

Questions 1–5	Answers
1. What is the rate?	Usually 40–60 beats per minute
2. What is the rhythm?	Usually regular; irregular if isolated junctional escape beat is present
3. Is there a P wave before each QRS? Are the P waves upright and uniform?	Inverted or absent May appear before or after the QRS
4. What is the length of the PR interval?	Usually less than 0.12 second if P wave precedes QRS; absent if no P wave occurs before QRS
5. Do all the QRS complexes look alike? What is the length of the QRS complexes?	Yes Less than 0.12 second (3 small squares)

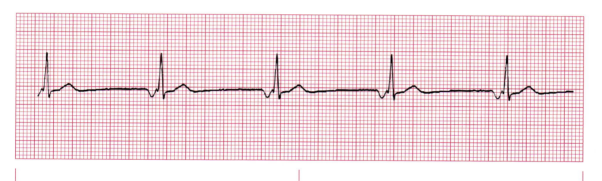

Figure 9–2.   Junctional escape rhythm

We generally refer to rhythms as **tachycardic** when the rate exceeds 100 bpm. In comparison with the intrinsic rate of the AV junction (40–60 bpm), the rate of this rhythm is generally around 60–100 bpm, thus the term "accelerated." When the junctional firing rate exceeds 100 bpm, the resulting rhythm is called **junctional tachycardia;** we will discuss this rhythm in the next section of this chapter. As you may now realize, description of the junctional rhythms is, in part, specific to the rate of impulse generation from the AV junction.

Causes of accelerated junctional rhythms include ischemia of the AV junction, hypoxia, digitalis intoxication, inferior wall myocardial infarction, and rheumatic fever. As with any dysrhythmia, and especially if symptoms are present, the patient should be carefully monitored.

You should, at this time, ask and answer the five questions that apply to interpreting an EKG rhythm strip. (See Table 9–3 and Figure 9–3.) Remember to apply each question slowly and methodically to the strip that you are observing in order to gain a complete understanding of the interpretation of the rhythm. Remember that memorization of strips **does not work** and will often lead you down the path to incorrect analysis. If in doubt, start over and ask the five questions again.

Remember that the rate of an accelerated junctional rhythm (60–100 bpm) will be greater than the intrinsic rate of the AV junction (40–60 bpm) and the P waves may be inverted or absent or occur after the QRS complexes. **Remember: Always monitor your patient's clinical condition!**

junctional tachycardia when the junctional firing rate exceeds 100 bpm

Table 9–3

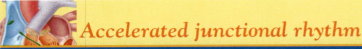

Accelerated junctional rhythm

Questions 1–5	Answers
1. What is the rate?	60–100 beats per minute
2. What is the rhythm?	Atrial: regular Ventricular: regular
3. Is there a P wave before each QRS? Are the P waves upright and uniform?	Inverted or absent May appear before or after the QRS
4. What is the length of the PR interval?	Usually less than 0.12 second if P wave precedes QRS; absent if no P wave occurs before QRS
5. Do all the QRS complexes look alike? What is the length of the QRS complexes?	Yes Less than 0.12 second (3 small squares)

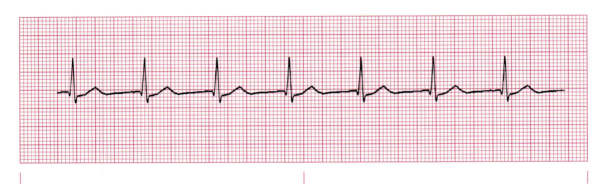

Figure 9–3. Accelerated junctional rhythm

JUNCTIONAL TACHYCARDIA RHYTHMS

junctional tachycardia rhythm a rhythm arising from the AV junctional tissue at a rate of 100–180 bpm

paroxysmal rhythm a rhythm observed to start or end abruptly

paroxysmal junctional tachycardia (PJT) rhythm a junctional tachycardia rhythm that is observed to begin or end abruptly

In our discussion of accelerated junctional rhythm, we determined that increased automaticity in the AV junction may cause the pacemaker cells of the junction to discharge impulses at a rate faster than its intrinsic rate. We also noted that rates exceeding 100 bpm are referred to as tachycardic. Assimilating these two facts, we now recognize that a rhythm arising from the AV junctional tissue at a rate of 100–180 bpm is referred to as a **junctional tachycardia rhythm.**

In our discussion of the atrial rhythms (Chapter 8), we determined that a rhythm observed to start or end abruptly is referred to as a **paroxysmal rhythm.** Thus a junctional tachycardia rhythm that is **observed** to begin or end abruptly is correctly called a **paroxysmal junctional tachycardia (PJT) rhythm.** Due to the rapid rate of a paroxysmal junctional tachycardia rhythm, it may be indistinguishable from other supraventricular tachycardic rhythms. Consequently, PJT may simply, and correctly, be referred to as a PSVT rhythm.

Causes of junctional tachycardia rhythms may include underlying ischemic heart disease, frequent ingestion of stimulants, anxiety, hypoxia, or rheumatic heart disease. An interesting aspect of PJT is that this rhythm may occur at any age, in a patient with no history of underlying cardiac disease. As with other dysrhythmias, treat-

Table 9–4

Junctional tachycardia

Questions 1–5	Answers
1. What is the rate?	100–180 beats per minute
2. What is the rhythm?	Atrial: regular Ventricular: regular
3. Is there a P wave before each QRS? Are the P waves upright and uniform?	If visible, inverted May appear before or after the QRS
4. What is the length of the PR interval?	Usually less than 0.12 second if P wave precedes QRS; absent if no P wave occurs before QRS
5. Do all the QRS complexes look alike? What is the length of the QRS complexes?	Yes Less than 0.12 second (3 small squares)

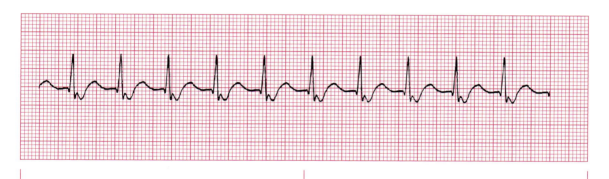

Figure 9–4.   Junctional tachycardia rhythm

ment (if indicated) is aimed at identifying and treating the underlying cause of the dysrhythmia.

Let's now apply the five-step approach to rhythm analysis to understand junctional tachycardia. (See Table 9–4 and Figure 9–4.)

Remember that the rate of a junctional tachycardia rhythm will be greater than 100 bpm. The P waves may be inverted (if visible) or absent or may occur after the QRS complexes. **Remember: Always monitor your patient's clinical condition!**

CLINICAL SIGNIFICANCE OF JUNCTIONAL RHYTHMS

Premature junctional contractions

The clinical significance of PJCs is based on the frequency of their occurrence and, most important, on the patient's clinical condition. Normally, isolated PJCs are of minimal significance. If PJCs are frequent (more than six per minute), you should recognize that more serious dysrhythmias may develop. In addition, frequent PJCs may signify underlying organic heart disease. Typically, management of patients who present with isolated PJCs includes only close observation.

Junctional escape rhythm

The clinical significance of junctional escape rhythms is based on the patient's heart rate and clinical condition. We know that the intrinsic rate of the AV junctional tissue is 40–60 bpm. If the patient's heart rate is nearer the lower end of the range, it is wise to be concerned with the possibility of decreased cardiac output. Decreased cardiac output may precipitate angina.

Patients may exhibit signs and symptoms of decreased perfusion, such as altered mental status, dizziness, and decreased blood pressure (hypotension). Treatment may include the administration of oxygen, as well as the consideration of atropine administration (or treatment per local protocols). If however, the rate is nearer 50–60 bpm, the junctional escape rhythm may be well tolerated.

Accelerated junctional rhythm

Accelerated junctional rhythm is generally well tolerated by the patient and usually requires no immediate intervention. In dealing with patients who are taking the drug digoxin, accelerated junctional rhythm may suggest the possibility of digitalis toxicity. Because ischemia is one possible cause of this rhythm, the patient must be carefully monitored for the occurrence of other, more serious dysrhythmias.

Junctional tachycardia rhythm

In a young patient with a healthy heart, junctional tachycardia may be well tolerated. This is not the case, however, in patients with cardiac compromise. Patients may report that they feel as though the heart is "running away" or "fluttering." Cardiac output may be significantly decreased, due to inadequate ventricular filling time. Sustained episodes of junctional tachycardia, especially at the high-rate range (160–180 bpm), may precipitate angina, congestive heart failure, pronounced hypoxia, or hypotension. Treatment is based on the patient's clinical appearance, signs, and symptoms and may include vagal maneuvers, drug therapy, and electrical therapy.

SUMMARY

Rhythms that are initiated in the area of the AV junction are called junctional rhythms. It will be helpful for you to recognize that all junctional dysrhythmias contain several similar EKG features. These common features include P waves that are inverted or absent, a PR interval that is usually less than 0.12 second in duration, and QRS complexes that are within normal limits. Typically, management of patients who present with junctional rhythms includes only close observation.

Review Questions
CHAPTER 9

1. The AV node is located in the:
   a. Right atrium
   b. Left ventricle
   c. Purkinje fiber tract
   d. Intraventricular septum

2. The intrinsic firing rate of the AV node is _____ minutes.
   a. 15–25
   b. 25–35
   c. 35–45
   d. 40–60

3. The intrinsic rate of the SA node in an adult is _____ minutes.
   a. 20–60
   b. 40–80
   c. 60–100
   d. 80–100

4. The treatment of uncomplicated acute myocardial infarction usually includes:
   a. IV D5W
   b. Oxygen by mask, IV LR
   c. IV NS, monitor, O2 via nasal cannula
   d. IV NS, monitor, O2, thrombolytic therapy

5. The chambers of the heart that are thin-walled and pump against low pressure are the:
   a. Apex
   b. Aorta
   c. Atria
   d. Ventricles

6. To distinguish PJT from sinus tachycardia, recall that a usual EKG feature of PJT is a _____ rate.
   a. More rapid
   b. Less rapid
   c. Less irregular
   d. More irregular

7. Rhythms that are _____ develop above the ventricles.

   a. Superventricular

   b. Idioventricular

   c. Supraventricular

   d. Retroventricular

8. PJCs resemble:

   a. PVCs

   b. PATs

   c. PACs

   d. PSVT

9. The rate of junctional tachycardia rhythms must be greater than _____ bpm.

   a. 200

   b. 100

   c. 300

   d. 260

10. When interpreting junctional rhythms, you should realize that the P waves may be:

    a. Inverted

    b. Absent

    c. Hidden in the QRS

    d. Any of the above

11. Premature junctional contractions (or complexes) are less common than premature atrial complexes (PACs) or premature ventricular contractions (PVCs).

    a. True

    b. False

12. Causes of PJCs may include:

    a. Fever

    b. Anxiety

    c. Drug effects

    d. All of the above

13. Myocardial ischemia can precipitate PJCs.

    a. True

    b. False

14.   PJCs may occur without any definite underlying cause.

    a.   True

    b.   False

15.   It is important to note that isolated occurrences of PJCs are not life-threatening.

    a.   True

    b.   False

Review Strips   CHAPTER 9

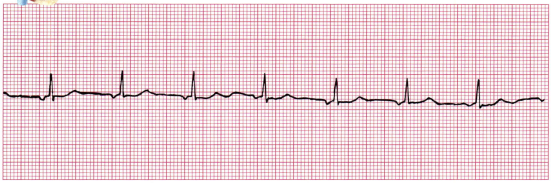

1. Rate _____   Rhythm _____
   P wave_____   PR interval_____
   QRS complex _____   Interpretation _____

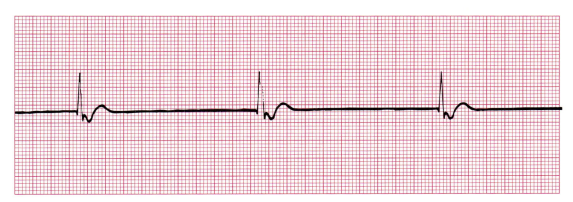

2. Rate _____   Rhythm _____
   P wave_____   PR interval_____
   QRS complex _____   Interpretation _____

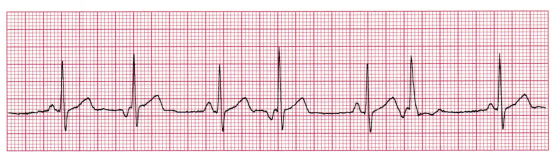

3. Rate _____ Rhythm _____

   P wave_____ PR interval_____

   QRS complex _____ Interpretation _____

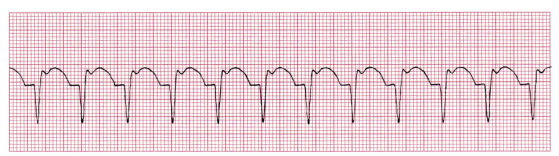

4. Rate _____ Rhythm _____

   P wave_____ PR interval_____

   QRS complex _____ Interpretation _____

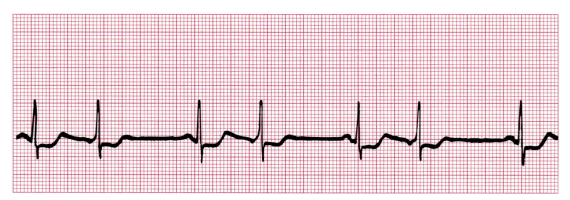

5. Rate _____ Rhythm _____

   P wave_____ PR interval_____

   QRS complex _____ Interpretation _____

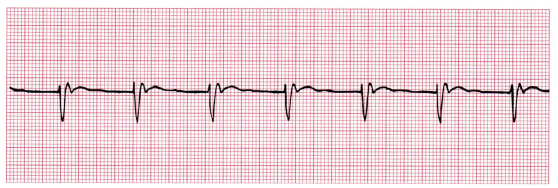

6. Rate _____   Rhythm _____

P wave_____   PR interval_____

QRS complex _____   Interpretation _____

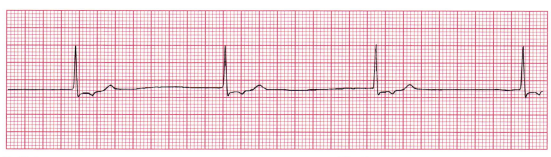

7. Rate _____   Rhythm _____

P wave_____   PR interval_____

QRS complex _____   Interpretation _____

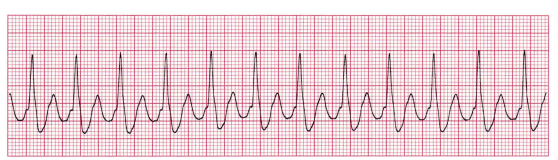

8. Rate _____   Rhythm _____

P wave_____   PR interval_____

QRS complex _____   Interpretation _____

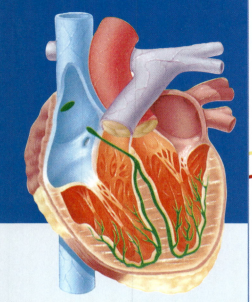

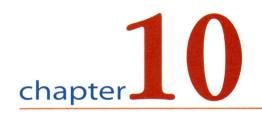

Introducing the Ventricular Rhythms

objectives

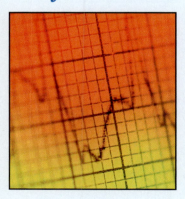

Upon completion of this chapter, the student will be able to:

➤ Discuss the origin of the ventricular rhythms

➤ Review specific components of the electrical conduction system of the heart

➤ Identify premature ventricular contractions, including EKG characteristics

➤ Identify idioventricular rhythm, including EKG characteristics

➤ Differentiate idioventricular rhythm and accelerated idioventricular rhythm

➤ Identify ventricular tachycardia, including EKG characteristics

➤ Identify ventricular fibrillation, including EKG characteristics

➤ Identify ventricular asystole, including EKG characteristics

➤ Discuss pulseless electrical activity

➤ Discuss the clinical significance of the ventricular rhythms

INTRODUCTION

In previous chapters, we have discussed rhythms that originate above the ventricles, or supraventricular rhythms. In this chapter, we will explore rhythms that have their origin in the ventricles. Ventricular rhythms are characteristically considered more dangerous than supraventricular rhythms. Despite this broad statement, it is imperative to remember that the significance of **any** rhythm is based on your patient's clinical condition.

REVIEW OF THE HEART'S ELECTRICAL CONDUCTION SYSTEM

In Chapter 8, we learned that the electrical activity produced by the conduction system of the heart is recorded as waveforms on EKG paper. Recall that the SA node is the usual, or expected, site of impulse generation. The electrical impulse leaves the SA node at a rate of 60–100 beats per minute (bpm) and travels through the atria via the internodal pathways, resulting in atrial depolarization. The AV node then receives and slows the impulse before allowing it to travel on through the AV junction, the bundle of His, and the left and right bundle branches, and down through the Purkinje fibers in the ventricles, causing ventricular depolarization. Although we know now that this is the normal route of impulses through the electrical conduction system, we have also learned that many variations can occur. One group of variations is called **ventricular dysrhythmias.**

ORIGIN OF VENTRICULAR RHYTHMS

Recall now that the pacemaker cells in the ventricles can, in certain instances, serve as the heart's pacemaker. An electrical impulse can be initiated from any pacemaker cell in the ventricles, including the bundle branches or the fibers of the Purkinje network.

When the SA node or the AV junctional tissues fail to initiate an electrical impulse, the ventricles will take the responsibility of pacing the heart. Think now about the intrinsic firing rate of the three pacemaker sites and review Table 10–1.

A brief review of this table clearly reminds you that the heart rate is significantly decreased when the ventricles assume the responsibility of pacing the heart. Remembering the relationship between heart rate and cardiac output immediately alerts us to the fact that cardiovascular compromise is a very real consideration when the ventricles are acting as the pacemaker of the heart. It is safe to say that the ventricles are the least efficient of the heart's pacemakers. This knowledge alone will alert us to the fact that the patient must be even more carefully monitored when the EKG strip or cardiac monitor demonstrates the attributes of a ventricular rhythm.

Table 10–1

Intrinsic firing rates of pacemaker sites

Sinoatrial (SA) Node	60–100 bpm
Atrioventricular (AV) junctional tissue	40–60 bpm
Purkinje network	20–40 bpm

Impulses that are ventricular in origin begin in the lower ventricular musculature. Hence the impulse may travel in a retrograde (backward) direction in order to depolarize the atria. Depending upon the actual **site of** origin, the impulse may travel antegrade (forward) to depolarize the ventricles. In either direction of travel, the normal conduction pathway is bypassed. Because of this bypass, ventricular rhythms will display QRS complexes that are wide (greater than or equal to 0.12 second) and bizarre in appearance, and P waves will be absent. P waves are indistinguishable because they are buried or hidden in the QRS complex. Remember that the QRS complexes of supraventricular rhythms are commonly less than 0.12 second in duration.

PREMATURE VENTRICULAR COMPLEXES (CONTRACTIONS)

In the initial discussion of premature ventricular complexes (PVCs), it is important to note that PVCs are individual complexes **rather than** an actual Rhythm. In your future studies of premature beats, you will undoubtedly find references to premature beats as "contractions" rather than complexes. It is wise, however, to realize that the more correct term to be used in the discussion of these premature beats is "complex," not "contraction."

A single, ectopic (out-of-place) complex that occurs earlier than the next expected complex and arises from an irritable site in the ventricles is referred to as a **premature ventricular complex.** Premature ventricular complexes are quite common occurrences and can appear in many heart rhythms. The significance of the appearance of PVCs is based entirely upon the patient's clinical condition.

Most commonly, the underlying cadence of the SA node is not interrupted by the occurrence of a PVC, nor is the SA node depolarized by the PVC. A premature ventricular complex is usually followed by a compensatory pause. Recall our earlier discussions regarding compensatory and noncompensatory pauses. You will remember that a compensatory pause is one in which the SA node is unaffected, nor is the cadence of the heart interrupted. The presence of *a compensatory pause*, coupled with a wide, bizarre, and premature QRS complex, is a highly suggestive indicator of PVCs.

On occasion, a PVC may fall between two sinus beats without interfering with the rhythm. This beat is referred to as an **interpolated beat.** As you are about to learn, PVCs may appear in many different patterns and shapes. Perhaps it is because of their bizarre appearance that PVCs are usually easier to discern than other premature beats.

The **morphology,** or shape, of the PVC is based on the site of origin of the ectopic focus. PVCs that are alike in appearance are called **unifocal**, while those with different shapes are called **multifocal.** Unifocal PVCs arise from one single site within the ventricles, whereas multifocal PVCs originate from different sites within the ventricles. Because PVCs often indicate myocardial irritability, you should note that multifocal PVCs are more serious than unifocal PVCs. If, for instance, you note an EKG strip containing PVCs with three or four different shapes, it should occur to you that there may be three or four different irritable sites within the ventricles. Any indication of increased myocardial irritability dictates that the patient should be carefully evaluated and managed, without delay. PVCs may be classified based on the basis of their frequency of occurrence, as illustrated in Table 10–2.

We should note here that there should be at least three episodes in a row on the monitor or EKG strip in order to correctly identify patterns of ventricular bigeminy, trigeminy, or quadrigeminy. Another name given to a run or grouping of 3 or more PVCs in a row (ventricular tachycardia, or VT, which is discussed later in this chapter) is **salvos.**

Because the terms that identify patterns of occurrences of PVCs can also be applied to PACs and PJCs, it may be wise to note the site of origin when identifying premature beats. In other words, rather than simply stating "bigeminy," a more correct interpreta-

premature ventricular complex a single, ectopic (out-of-place) complex that occurs earlier than the next expected complex and arises from an irritable site in the ventricles

interpolated beat occurs when a PVC falls between two sinus beats without interfering with the rhythm

morphology shape of the PVC

unifocal PVCs that are alike in appearance

multifocal PVCs with different shapes that originate from different sites within the ventricles

salvos another name given to a run or grouping of 3 or more PVCs in a row

Table 10–2

PVC patterns of occurrence

Ventricular bigeminy	Occurs when every other beat is a PVC
Ventricular trigeminy	Occurs when every third beat is a PVC
Ventricular quadrigeminy	Occurs when every fourth beat is a PVC
Couplet or repetitive PVCs	Two PVCs occurring together without a normal complex inbetween
Runs of ventricular tachycardia (VT)	Three or more PVCs in a row

tion might be "ventricular bigeminy." Again, it's better to add a millisecond in time to your rhythm interpretation than to risk the possibility of an incorrect interpretation.

Test yourself by asking why ventricular bigeminy, couplets, and runs of ventricular tachycardia are very significant rhythm presentations. You should have answered the question by recalling that these particular rhythms tend to indicate increased myocardial irritability and may be precursors of more serious, perhaps lethal, dysrhythmias. This is even more notable if the PVCs happen to occur during the relative refractory, or vulnerable, period, during repolarization. Premature ventricular complexes are considered particularly dangerous if they occur more than six times in a one-minute EKG strip (frequent PVCs), if they occur in couplets or runs of VT, or if they occur in a patient who is hemodynamically unstable.

Premature ventricular complexes are also considered very dangerous if they fall on the T wave of the preceding beat (R-on-T phenomenon). If you recall our earlier discussion of the refractory periods, you will understand that the myocardium is in its most vulnerable state (electrically) during this period. A PVC that falls on the T wave may thus trigger repetitious ventricular contractions, resulting in ventricular fibrillation.

Causes of premature ventricular complexes include myocardial irritability (due to **myocardial ischemia**), increased emotional stress or physical exertion, congestive heart failure, electrolyte imbalances, digitalis toxicity, or acid-base imbalances. It is important to note that PVCs may also occur as simply a normal variant in some individuals. Treatment of PVCs, as with all dysrhythmias, is based on the patient's clinical symptoms and may range from oxygen to pharmaceutical antidysrhythmics.

Let's now apply the five-step approach to investigate the rules for interpretation of PVCs. (See Table 10–3 and Figures 10–1 through 10–6.)

myocardial ischemia
decreased supply of oxygenated blood to the heart

Table 10–3

Premature ventricular complexes

Questions 1–5	Answers
1. What is the rate?	Dependent on rate of underlying rhythm and number of PVCs
2. What is the rhythm?	Occasionally irregular; regular if interpolated PVC
3. Is there a P wave before each QRS? Are the P waves upright and uniform?	No P waves associated with PVC P waves of underlying rhythm may be present
4. What is the length of the PR interval?	PRI not present with PVCs
5. What do the QRS complexes look like? The length of the QRS complexes is:	Equal to or greater than 0.12 second (3 small squares); usually wide and bizarre

Remember that the number of PVCs is included in the total count of R waves in calculating the rate in rhythms containing PVCs. One key in the recognition of PVCs is the usual wide, bizarre appearance of the QRS. **Remember: Always monitor your patient's clinical condition!**

IDIOVENTRICULAR RHYTHM

idioventricular rhythms (IVRs) (also called ventricular escape rhythms) result when the discharge rate of higher pacemakers become less than that of the ventricles or when impulses from higher pacemakers fail to reach the ventricles

Idioventricular rhythms (IVRs) are also called *ventricular escape rhythms* and are considered a last-ditch effort of the ventricles to try to prevent cardiac standstill. The appearance of this rhythm most commonly indicates that the SA node and the AV junctional tissue have failed to function as pacemakers or that the rate of these higher pacemakers has fallen below the intrinsic rate of the ventricles. Neither P waves nor PR intervals are produced, because the atria do not depolarize. Although ventricular depolarization does occur, the rate is usually less than 40 beats per minute and cardiac output is usually compromised.

agonal when the rate of an IVR rhythm falls below 20 bpm, the rhythm may be called agonal

When the rate of an IVR rhythm falls below 20 bpm, the rhythm may be called **agonal.** Agonal rhythm may frequently be seen as the last ordered semblance of heart rhythm when a resuscitation attempt has been unsuccessful. Idioventricular rhythm may commonly be seen as the first organized rhythm following successful defibrillation. Causes of IVR include extensive myocardial damage, secondary to acute myocardial infarction, or failure of higher pacemakers. IVR is considered a lethal rhythm, and treatment must be immediate and aggressive.

Although the absence of P waves and the widened QRS complexes on the EKG strip are obvious, it is wise to follow your basic five-step approach in the interpretation of this rhythm (Table 10–4).

Recognize that an idioventricular rhythm is an ominous sign. **It is critical that you remember to monitor your patient's clinical condition closely.**

accelerated idioventricular rhythm (AIVR) occurs when the rate of the ectopic pacemaker in an idioventricular rhythm exceeds 40 beats per minute

ACCELERATED IDIOVENTRICULAR RHYTHM

An **accelerated idioventricular rhythm (AIVR)** may occur when the rate of the ectopic pacemaker in an idioventricular rhythm exceeds 40 beats per minute. The commonly accepted rate of AIVR is 40–100 beats per minute. Because the atria do not

Table 10–4

Idioventricular rhythm

Questions 1–5	Answers
1. What is the rate?	20–40 beats per minute or less
2. What is the rhythm?	Atrial rhythm not distinguishable; ventricular rhythm usually regular
3. Is there a P wave before each QRS?	No; none present
4. What is the length of the PR interval?	None
5. Do all the QRS complexes look alike? What is the length of the QRS complexes?	Yes; bizarre morphology Greater than 0.12 second

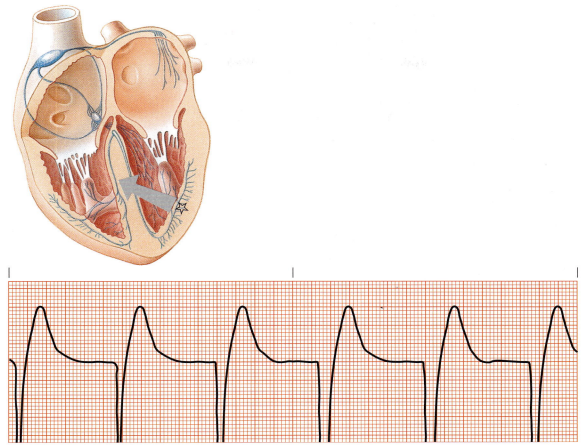

Figure 10–7.   Accelerated idioventricular rhythm

depolarize, there are no P waves or PR intervals noted on an EKG strip that depicts AIVR (see Figure 10–7).

Accelerated idioventricular rhythm may occur in conjunction with myocardial ischemia. Because of the morphology of the QRS complexes in ventricular dysrhythmias, it is very important that the heart rate be carefully evaluated. Accelerated idioventricular rhythm can be mistaken for ventricular tachycardia unless there is a careful assessment of the patient and the patient's heart rate. As noted earlier, the usual rate of an AIVR is 40–100 bpm; the rate of ventricular tachycardia is usually greater than 120 bpm. Although experts and various references may disagree on **exact** ranges of heart rates of ventricular dysrhythmias, it is imperative to *remember that you must always assess and treat the patient, <u>rather</u> than the monitor or EKG strip.*

VENTRICULAR TACHYCARDIA

The most commonly accepted definition of **ventricular tachycardia (VT or V tach)** describes this rhythm as one in which three or more PVCs arise in sequence at a rate of greater than 100 beats per minute. This rhythm commonly overrides the normal pacemaker of the heart.

ventricular tachycardia (VT or V tach) rhythm in which three or more PVCs arise in sequence at a rate of greater than 100 beats per minute; commonly overrides the normal pacemaker of the heart

Table 10–5

Ventricular tachycardia rhythm

Questions 1–5	Answers
1. What is the rate?	100–250 beats per minute
2. What is the rhythm?	Atrial rhythm not distinguishable; ventricular rhythm usually regular
3. Is there a P wave before each QRS?	May be present or absent; not associated with QRS complexes
4. What is the length of the PR interval?	None
5. Do all the QRS complexes look alike? What is the length of the QRS complexes?	Yes (except in torsades rhythm); bizarre QRS morphology Greater than 0.12 second

sustained rhythm a rhythm that lasts for more than 30 seconds

nonsustained rhythm a run of VT that lasts for less than 30 seconds

hemodynamically unstable refers to a patient who presents with hypotension (low blood pressure), chest pain, shortness of breath, and changes in mental status

hemodynamically stable refers to a patient who presents with a normal blood pressure (normotensive), absence of chest pain, and no notable change in mental status

Quite often, this dysrhythmia occurs rapidly and is initiated by a PVC or by PVCs occurring in rapid succession. If this rhythm is sustained, the patient's clinical condition may rapidly deteriorate. It is important to note that some patients may, in fact, tolerate a sustained V tach rhythm without immediate decompensation; however this is the exception, not the rule. A **sustained rhythm** is generally thought to be a rhythm that lasts for more than 30 seconds. If a run of VT lasts for less than 30 seconds, it is a **nonsustained rhythm,** or simply a run of V tach.

When a ventricular ectopic beat occurs at a rate of 100–250 beats per minute, ventricular tachycardia may result. P waves may be present if the SA node retains control of the atria; however, if P waves are present, they have no set relationship to the QRS complexes. PR intervals are not discernible. The QRS complexes in VT will appear wide and bizarre, measuring greater than 0.12 second in duration. The ventricular rhythm in VT is essentially regular.

Ventricular tachycardia is classified (on the basis of assessment of the patients' clinical presentation) as either **pulseless V tach** or **V tach with a pulse.** Immediate treatment for the patient who exhibits V tach on the monitor is based on the presence or absence of a palpable pulse. Pulseless ventricular tachycardia is treated as ventricular fibrillation, with immediate defibrillation.

The treatment of V tach with a pulse is based on the patient's clinical picture; thus you must assess whether the patient is stable or unstable. If the patient is hemodynamically unstable, immediate cardioversion is considered. If the patient is hemodynamically stable, drug intervention is appropriate.

"Hemodynamically unstable" refers to a patient who presents with hypotension (low blood pressure), chest pain, shortness of breath, and changes in mental status. The change in mental status may signal a decrease in cerebral perfusion. A patient who is **hemodynamically stable** will usually present with a normal blood pressure (normotensive), absence of chest pain, and no notable change in mental status.

Causes of ventricular tachycardia are somewhat synonymous with the causes of PVCs. These causes include myocardial ischemia, hypoxia, electrolyte imbalances, increased anxiety or physical exertion, and underlying heart disease. Consider the key points regarding interpretation of V tach as you perform your five-step approach to the rhythm represented in Table 10–5 and Figure 10–8.

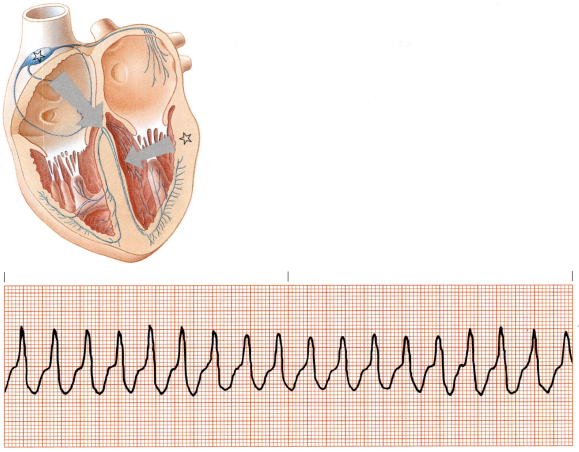

Figure 10–8.   Ventricular tachycardia

Remember that ventricular tachycardia is a potentially life-threatening dysrhythmia. It is vital that you **remember to monitor your patient's clinical condition closely.**

TORSADES DE POINTES

A rhythm that is similar to ventricular tachycardia is **torsades de pointes.** This name is derived from a French term meaning "twisting of the points." The morphology of QRS complexes in a torsades rhythm show variations in width and shape. This rhythm resembles a turning about or a twisting motion along the baseline (isoelectric line). This life-threatening dysrhythmia may result from hypokalemia, hypomagnesemia, an overdose of a tricyclic antidepressant drug, the use of antidysrhythmic drugs, or a combination of these.

Although torsades is often responsive to electrical therapy, it is wise to remember that this dysrhythmia has an annoying tendency to recur repeatedly. Therefore, finding and treating the underlying cause of the rhythm is essential. Magnesium is the pharmacologic treatment of choice for torsades de pointes. Remember that the **key** to recognizing torsades is the variation of QRS morphology, or shape, as illustrated in Figure 10–9.

torsades de pointes similar to ventricular tachycardia; morphology of QRS complexes show variations in width and shape; life-threatening dysrhythmia

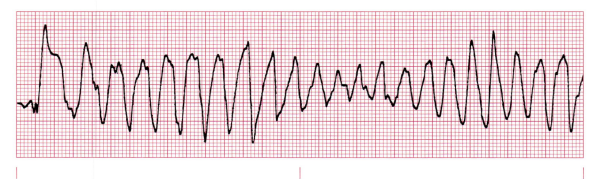

Figure 10–9. Torsades de pointes

VENTRICULAR FIBRILLATION

ventricular fibrillation (V fib, VF) is a fatal dysrhythmia that occurs as a result of multiple weak ectopic foci in the ventricles; there is no coordinated atrial or ventricular contraction and no palpable pulse

Ventricular fibrillation (V fib, VF) is a fatal dysrhythmia. Ventricular fibrillation is thought to be the most frequent initial rhythm occurrence in sudden cardiac arrest, according to the American Heart Association. Ventricular fibrillation tends to occur in the initial hours following an acute myocardial infarction.

This rhythm occurs as a result of multiple weak ectopic foci in the ventricles. There is no coordinated atrial or ventricular contraction and no palpable pulse. The myocardial cells appear to quiver rather than depolarize normally. In ventricular fibrillation, electrical impulses are initiated by multiple ventricular sites; however, these impulses are not transmitted through the normal conduction pathway. There are, therefore, no usual waveforms apparent on the EKG strip or monitor.

The waveforms in ventricular fibrillation appear as disorganized, rapid, irregular waves whose morphology vary vastly. There are no well-organized QRS complexes. Because no blood is being circulated throughout the body, death will occur if immediate treatment is not established.

Ventricular fibrillation is further classified as either *fine ventricular fibrillation or coarse ventricular fibrillation.* These two types of VF can be defined on the basis of amplitude (height) of VF waves. Ventricular fibrillation waves of less than 3 millimeters' amplitude are described as *fine.* Ventricular fibrillation waves with amplitudes greater than 3 millimeters are considered *coarse.* Coarse VF waves are generally more irregular than fine VF waves. Coarse VF will progress to fine VF unless treatment is initiated in a timely manner. It is notable to add that coarse VF responds better than fine VF to treatment (electrical therapy).

Thorough patient assessment is critical, because artifact or loose leads can closely resemble ventricular fibrillation. Look at your patient and always, always <u>treat the patient, not the monitor</u>. If your patient is sitting up in bed, reading a newspaper, or conversing with you in a coherent manner, chances are **very good** that he or she is not experiencing ventricular fibrillation!

Causes of ventricular fibrillation include acute myocardial infarction, myocardial ischemia, drug toxicity or overdose, hypoxia, coronary artery disease, and a variety of other causes. Regardless of the cause of ventricular fibrillation, prompt intervention is vital to the survival of your patient.

As you review Table 10–6 and Figure 10–10 while applying the five-step approach, you may realize that the absence of waveforms indicates the absence of life-sustaining myocardial function.

Table 10–6

Ventricular fibrillation

Questions 1–5	Answers
1. What is the rate?	Rate cannot be discerned
2. What is the rhythm?	Rapid, unorganized rhythm not distinguishable
3. Is there a P wave before each QRS?	No
4. What is the length of the PR interval?	None present
5. Do all the QRS complexes look alike? What is the length of the QRS complexes?	None present

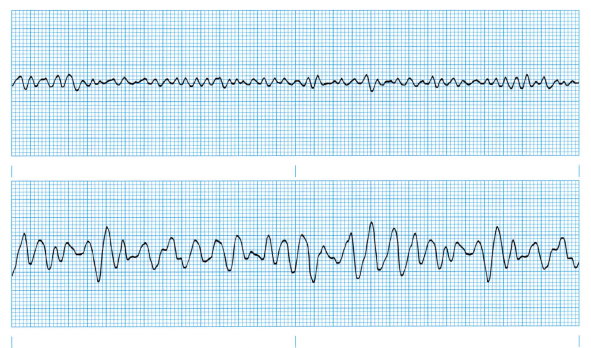

Figure 10–10.   Ventricular fibrillation (fine and coarse)

Remember that ventricular fibrillation is a life-threatening dysrhythmia and will result in death unless immediate treatment is initiated. **Monitor your patient's clinical condition closely.**

ASYSTOLE OR VENTRICULAR ASYSTOLE

The absence of all ventricular activity is known as **ventricular asystole.** Ventricular asystole is also called **cardiac standstill** or **asystole**. The technical, or literal, definition of asystole is the absence of all cardiac electrical activity. However, the terms are sometimes used interchangeably. Asystole is represented by a flat line (consistent with the isoelectric line on an EKG strip). Actually, asystole is not a rhythm; it represents the absence of all electrical activity and is indicative of clinical death (the absence of pulse and respirations).

ventricular asystole the absence of all ventricular activity; also called cardiac standstill or asystole; the absence of all cardiac electrical activity

Table 10–7

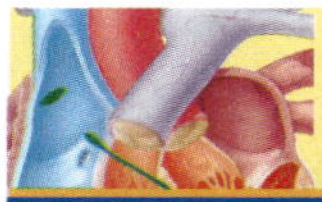

Ventricular asystole	
Questions 1–5	**Answers**
1. What is the rate?	Absent
2. What is the rhythm?	Absent Rhythm not distinguishable
3. Is there a P wave before each QRS?	No
4. What is the length of the PR interval?	None present
5. Do all the QRS complexes look alike? What is the length of the QRS complexes?	None present

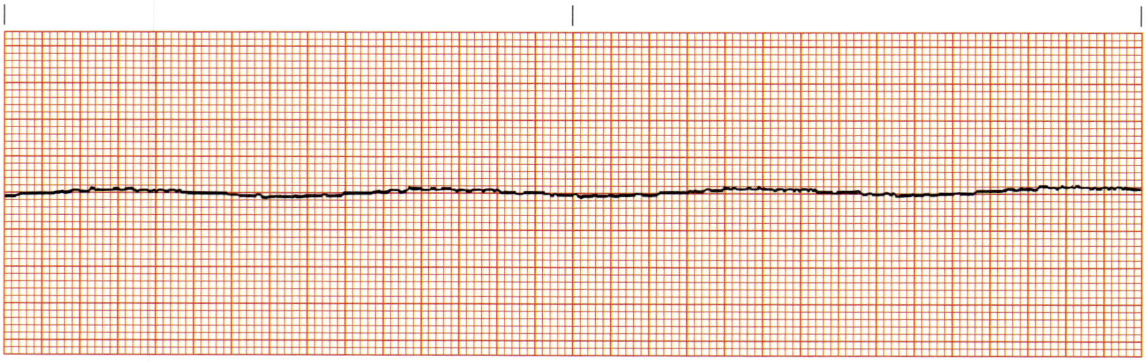

Figure 10–11.   Ventricular asystole (cardiac standstill, asystole)

The most notable characteristic of asystole is the total absence of waveforms on an EKG strip or cardiac monitor. It may be difficult to distinguish asystole from very fine VF; therefore, you must always check two different leads (e.g., Lead II and Lead III) in order to identify asystole definitively.

Asystole often follows unsuccessful resuscitation attempts. It may be caused by massive myocardial infarction, cardiac trauma, ventricular aneurysm, and complete heart block. Ventricular asystole may often be the initial event in cardiac arrest.

In your application of the five-step approach to dysrhythmia interpretation, you will note that the rhythm in Table 10–7 and Figure 10–11 indicates the absence of both mechanical and electrical cardiac activity.

Resuscitation attempts are often unsuccessful, and the prognosis for patients who present with asystole is poor. Ventricular asystole is a terminal dysrhythmia and will result in death unless immediate treatment is initiated. **Closely monitor the patient's clinical condition!**

PULSELESS ELECTRICAL ACTIVITY

pulseless electrical activity (PEA) the absence of a palpable pulse and myocardial muscle activity with the presence of organized electrical activity (excluding VT or VF) on the cardiac monitor

The absence of a palpable pulse and myocardial muscle activity with the presence of organized electrical activity (excluding VT or VF) on the cardiac monitor is called **pulseless electrical activity (PEA).** Pulseless electrical activity is not an actual rhythm; rather, it represents a clinical condition wherein the patient is clinically dead, despite the fact that some type of organized rhythm appears on the monitor. PEA was formerly called electromechanical dissociation, EMD. Like asystole, this rhythm conveys a grave prognosis.

Causes of PEA include profound hypovolemia, massive myocardial damage, ventricular rupture, pulmonary embolism, acidosis, and massive cardiac trauma, which may result in cardiac tamponade or tension pneumothorax. The underlying cause or causes of PEA must be rapidly identified and treated in order for the patient to survive.

CLINICAL SIGNIFICANCE OF VENTRICULAR DYSRHYTHMIAS

Premature Ventricular Complexes

Premature ventricular complexes may be of little or no significance in patients who have no history of heart disease. These patients may report a feeling of "skipped beats," and some patients will refer to the extra beats as **"palpitations."** Patients may even relate that their intake of caffeine or their level of stress has increased recently. From previous experience, patients will often report that the "skipped beats" seemed to disappear when they reduced their intake of stimulants or their level of stress. This seems a good time to remind you that listening, *truly listening,* to your patients can be one of the most valuable assessment tools available to you.

palpitations a sensation that the heart is skipping beats and/or beating rapidly

If your patient presents with evidence of myocardial ischemia (chest pain, anxiety, shortness of breath) and is exhibiting PVCs on the monitor or EKG strip, your index of suspicion should be heightened. Recall now that PVCs can indicate varying degrees of ventricular irritability and may be followed by more serious dysrhythmias. In addition, it is wise to remember that cardiac output may be compromised if PVCs are frequent. Recall the patterns of PVCs that are considered dangerous or "warning signs," and be alert for the occurrence of these patterns. Keep in mind that, often, the administration of oxygen may abate the PVCs. Most important, assess your patient's overall clinical picture. *Treat the patient, not the monitor!*

Idioventricular rhythm

The majority of patients who present with an idioventricular rhythm will be symptomatic. This is more easily understood when you recall that the heart rate is often slowed significantly with idioventricular rhythms. Cardiac compromise is always a concern in a patient with a slow heart rate. As a direct result of the decreased heart rate (bradycardia) and in conjunction with a decrease in cardiac output, the patient may present with weakness, dizziness, severe hypotension, and alterations in mental status.

It is essential that a thorough patient assessment be conducted in order to determine whether the rhythm is perfusing (producing a palpable pulse) or nonperfusing (signifying pulseless electrical activity). In instances of accelerated idioventricular rhythm, treatment is not indicated unless the patient is symptomatic.

Ventricular tachycardia

Ventricular tachycardia may be perfusing (producing a palpable pulse) or nonperfusing (producing no palpable pulse). Because of the rapid heart rate in V tach, the ventricles do not have time to adequately empty and refill; thus cardiac output will be compromised.

Recall that cardiac compromise can lead to decreased cerebral and myocardial perfusion because of inadequate amounts of blood circulating through the body. Treatment of V tach is based on the absence or presence of a palpable pulse, as well as the patient's clinical picture.

If the patient in V tach is perfusing and stable, treatment may consist of oxygen, administration, implementation of an IV lifeline, and pharmacologic intervention. If the patient is, or becomes, clinically unstable (as evidenced by marked hypotension, chest pain, and shortness of breath), synchronized cardioversion may be indicated. If the patient is unstable (nonperfusing), the immediate treatment will consist of unsynchronized cardioversion (defibrillation). Remember that pulseless V tach is treated as if it were ventricular fibrillation. The treatment must be aggressive and immediate.

Ventricular fibrillation

With ventricular fibrillation, there is no cardiac output, no perfusion, and no evidence of organized electrical activity in the heart. In other words, the patient is in cardiac arrest. If this rhythm is not treated immediately and aggressively, the patient will not be able to sustain life. Most cardiac arrests result from either ventricular tachycardia or ventricular fibrillation. The presence of fine V fib indicates that the rhythm has been present for an extended period of time. Treatment for ventricular fibrillation must be immediate and decisive. This treatment includes CPR, defibrillation (360 joules), airway control, IV lifeline, and drug intervention. The prognosis for patients with this life-threatening rhythm is less than encouraging. Nevertheless, the patient is treated aggressively, in order to give him or her every possible chance to survive.

Asystole

Ventricular asystole signals a complete termination of ventricular activity. Often asystole is considered a confirmation of death. Always remember to check the rhythm in two leads in order to rule out the possibility of the presence of fine V fib. If the rhythm appears to be fine V fib, it should be treated as V fib. Treatment of asystole, if attempted, includes CPR, placement of IV lifelines, endotracheal intubation, and pharmacologic intervention. Contrary to many popular television programs, defibrillation is not indicated with asystole! As with **all** dysrhythmias, treatment must always be based on conscientious and thorough patient assessment.

SUMMARY

The group of rhythms discussed in this chapter comprise the rhythms that are most commonly considered life-threatening. Ventricular rhythms often indicate myocardial ischemia and consequently must be diligently assessed and, where indicated, treated aggressively. In many instances, the outcome for the patient may depend upon the rapidity of recognition and treatment of ventricular dysrhythmias.

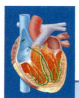

Review Questions
CHAPTER 10

1. PVCs characteristically have a _____ pause.
    a. Noncompensatory
    b. Uncompensatory
    c. Compensatory
    d. 0.30-second

2. The QRS complex corresponds to what electrical activity in the heart?
    a. Ventricular depolarization
    b. Atrial depolarization
    c. Ventricular contraction
    d. Atrial contraction

3. Pacemaker cells found in the Purkinje network in the ventricles have an intrinsic firing rate of _____ bpm.
    a. 20–30
    b. 60–80
    c. 40–60
    d. 20–40

4. Atrial activity is not discerned on an EKG strip in all of the following rhythms except:
    a. IVR
    b. AIVR
    c. A fib
    d. VT

5. Ventricular diastole refers to ventricular:
    a. Contraction
    b. Relaxation
    c. Systole
    d. Pressure ratio

6. The heart ventricle with the thickest myocardium is the:
    a. Right
    b. Left

7. The coronary arteries receive oxygenated blood from the:

   a. Aorta

   b. Coronary sinus

   c. Pulmonary veins

   d. Pulmonary arteries

8. The QRS interval should normally be _____ second or smaller.

   a. 0.20

   b. 0.12

   c. 0.18

   d. 0.36

9. Oscilloscopic evidence of ventricular fibrillation can be mimicked by artifact.

   a. True

   b. False

10. The neurotransmitter for the parasympathetic nervous system is acetylcholine. Release of acetylcholine:

    1. Slows the heart rate

    2. Increases the heart rate

    3. Slows atrioventricular conduction

    4. Increases atrioventricular conduction

    a. 1 and 3

    b. 2 and 3

    c. 3 and 4

    d. 1 and 4

11. The most notable characteristic of asystole is the total absence of waveforms on an EKG strip or cardiac monitor.

    a. True

    b. False

12. It may be difficult to distinguish asystole from very fine VF; therefore, you must always check _____ different leads in order to definitively identify asystole.

    a. Four

    b. Three

    c. Two

    d. Five

13. PEA is not an actual rhythm; rather, it represents a clinical condition wherein the patient is clinically dead, despite the fact that some type of organized rhythm appears on the monitor.

    a. True

    b. False

14. This rhythm resembles a turning about or twisting motion along the baseline (iso-electric line).

   a. Ventricular tachycardia

   b. Ventricular asystole

   c. Torsades de pointes

   d. Pulseless electrical activity

15. PEA, a life-threatening dysrhythmia, may result from:

   a. Hypokalemia

   b. Hypomagnesemia

   c. Tricyclic antidepressant drug overdose

   d. All of the above

 Review Strips **CHAPTER 10**

1. Rate _____   Rhythm _____
    P wave_____   PR interval_____
    QRS complex _____   Interpretation _____

2. Rate _____   Rhythm _____
    P wave_____   PR interval_____
    QRS complex _____   Interpretation _____

Table 11–1

First-degree AV block

Questions 1–5	Answers
1. What is the rate?	Based on the rate of the underlying rhythm
2. What is the rhythm?	Usually regular
3. Is there a P wave before each QRS? Are the P waves upright and uniform?	Yes Yes
4. What is the length of the PR interval?	Greater than 0.20 second (3–5 small squares)
5. Do all the QRS complexes look alike? What is the length of the QRS complexes?	Yes Less than 0.12 second (3 small squares)

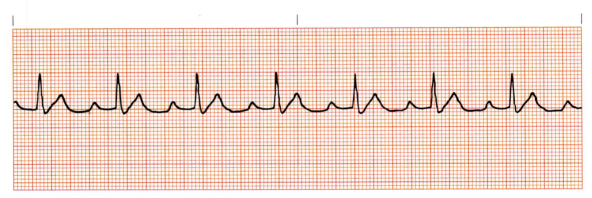

Figure 11–1. First-degree AV block

SECOND-DEGREE HEART BLOCKS

Now we will discuss the two types of **second-degree heart block.** The first type of the second degree blocks is less serious than the second type because bradycardia is less likely to be present and because cardiac output is less likely to be seriously decreased in a second-degree type I block.

The variety of names assigned to the two types of second-degree blocks are those of the two physicians who initially identified and described these heart blocks: Karel F. Wenckebach (1864), a Dutch-Austrian physician, and Woldemar Mobitz (1889), a German physician. Both were instrumental in the research, classification, and investigation of these two types of heart blocks.

Second-degree AV block (Mobitz Type I or Wenckebach)

The progressive prolongation of the electrical impulse delay at the AV node produces an increase in the length of the PR interval in **second-degree AV block.** A characteristic cyclic pattern is produced: the PR interval continues to increase in length until such time as the impulse is not conducted or a QRS complex is "dropped." This pattern is repetitive throughout the duration of the rhythm. Because of the "dropped" beat, the impulse does not reach the ventricles; therefore, ventricular contraction does not occur. The ventricular rhythm is irregular, but the atrial rhythm remains regular. Second-degree Mobitz type I heart block is also referred to as the Wenckebach phenomenon or simply Mobitz type I.

Mobitz I may be caused by abnormal conduction of the electrical impulses at the AV node and precipitated by AV node ischemia, digitalis therapy, or increased vagal

second-degree AV block, Mobitz type I, or Wenckenbach
the progressive prolongation of the electrical impulse delay at the AV node produces an increase in the length of the PR interval

Table 11–2

Second-degree block, Mobitz type I

Questions 1–5	Answers
1. What is the rate?	Atrial unaffected; ventricular rate is usually slower than atrial
2. What is the rhythm?	Atrial rhythm regular Ventricular rhythm irregular
3. Is there a P wave before each QRS? Are the P waves upright and uniform?	Yes Yes, for conducted beats
4. What is the length of the PR interval?	Progressively prolongs until a QRS is not conducted
5. Do all the QRS complexes look alike? What is the length of the QRS complexes?	Yes Less than 0.12 second

tone. It may also occur as a complication of an inferior myocardial infarction. Note that this rhythm is usually transient and will often resolve without outside intervention.

As you apply the five-step approach to analyze this rhythm, you should note the progressive prolongation of the PR interval until the point that the QRS complex does not appear (Table 11–2 and Figure 11–2).

Remember that a progressively prolonging PR interval is the **key** to recognizing second-degree Mobitz I heart block. **Remember: Always monitor your patient's clinical condition!**

Second-degree AV block (Mobitz Type II)

Second-degree AV block, or **Mobitz type II,** is a more serious dysrhythmia than either first-degree block or Mobitz type I. This is because type II indicates an increased risk of progression to third-degree, or complete, heart block. Mobitz type II occurs when there is an intermittent interruption in the electrical conduction system near or below the AV junction.

To understand this dysrhythmia, you should understand that the SA node is functionally unimpaired. In other words, the SA node is generating electrical impulses at regular intervals. Therefore, you should note that P waves will occur in a regular pattern across the EKG strip. You should also note, however, that some P waves are not followed by a QRS complex, because the impulse is completely blocked in one bundle branch and periodically blocked in the other bundle branch (these blocks are referred to as *bundle branch blocks*). We earlier referred to the AV node as the "gatekeeper" to the ventricles, so it may be helpful to remember now that in Mobitz type II the gate closes at regular intervals. When the gate closes, the impulse cannot be conducted through the bundle of His to the ventricles; thus no QRS complex is produced.

Second-degree blocks are often referred to by the ratio of P waves to QRS complexes. This ratio may vary or may be constant. The ratio of P waves to QRS complexes is often 2:1, 3:1, or 4:1. It may be easier to remember that an EKG strip of Mobitz type II may present as the appearance of two P waves for every QRS complex, three P waves for every QRS complex, or four P waves for every QRS complex.

Recall now that second-degree block, Mobitz II, represents a complete block of one of the bundle branches and a partial block of the other branch. It is because of this conduction disorder that the QRS complex will often be widened (greater than 0.12 second). Characteristically, this type of heart block will produce PR intervals that are regular in

second-degree AV block, or Mobitz type II a more serious dysrhythmia that occurs when there is an intermittent interruption in the electrical conduction system near or below the AV junction

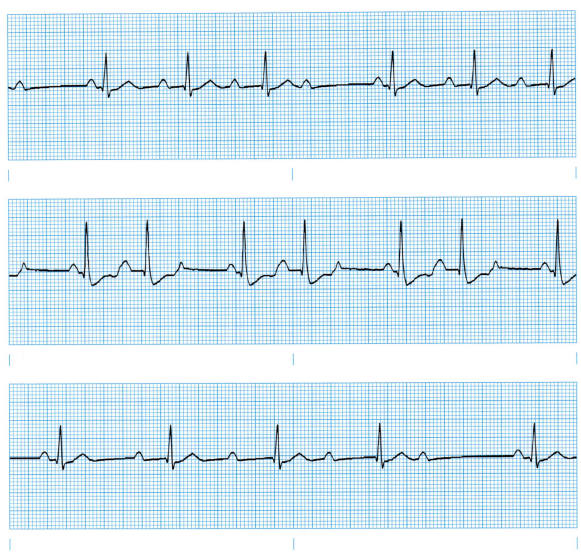

Figure 11–2. Second-degree heart block, Mobitz type I

length (for conducted beats), more P waves than QRS complexes, and a pattern that depicts intermittently absent QRS complexes.

It is important to note that the PR interval in Mobitz type II is constant, or regular, for every conducted beat. Recall that this occurs because the SA node is "firing" at a regular pace, but the impulse is blocked or is not allowed to be conducted at certain intervals. Whereas the atrial rhythm is regular, the ventricular rhythm is irregular because of the dropped or nonconducted beats.

Mobitz II may be associated with septal wall necrosis, acute myocardial infarction, acute myocarditis, or advanced coronary artery disease. Depending on the ventricular rate, the patient may be symptomatic or asymptomatic. If the ventricular rate is fast enough to sustain cardiac output at an effective level, the patient may not exhibit overt signs or symptoms. In this heart block, it is more common for the patient to exhibit signs or symptoms of decreased perfusion.

Review Table 11–3 and apply the five-step approach to the rhythm strips that follow (Figure 11–3). As you review the table and strip illustrations, consider the effect of a 2:1 block on cardiac output and overall perfusion.

Table 11–3

Second-degree block, Mobitz II

Questions 1–5	Answers
1. What is the rate?	Atrial rate regular; ventricular rate may be bradycardic
2. What is the rhythm?	Atrial rhythm regular Ventricular rhythm irregular
3. Is there a P wave before each QRS? Are the P waves upright and uniform?	Yes; some P waves are not followed by a QRS complex P waves are usually upright and uniform
4. What is the length of the PR interval?	Constant for conducted beats
5. Do all the QRS complexes look alike? What is the length of the QRS complexes?	Yes; intermittently absent less than or greater than 0.12 second

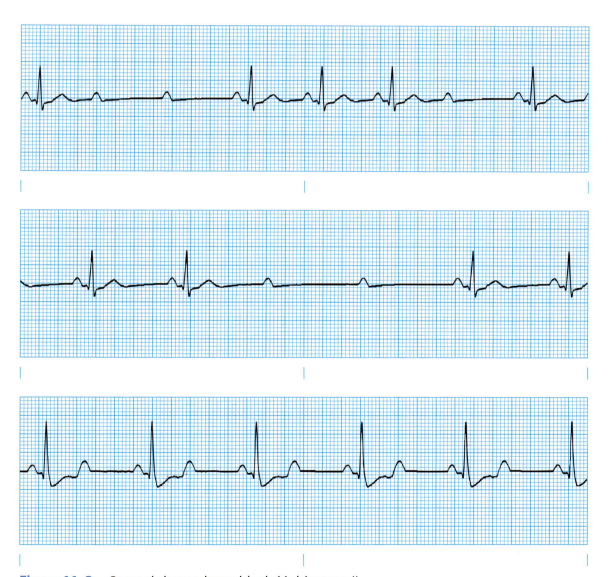

Figure 11–3. Second-degree heart block, Mobitz type II

Remember that the **keys** to interpreting Mobitz type II include the constancy of the PR intervals (for conducted beats) and intermittently absent QRS complexes. **Remember: Always monitor your patient's clinical condition!**

THIRD-DEGREE AV BLOCK (COMPLETE)

third-degree AV block (complete) the most serious type of heart block; the atria and ventricles are completely blocked or separated from each other electrically at or below the AV node; ventricular rate will most commonly be between 20 and 40 bpm

Third-degree heart block is, without question, the most serious type of heart block. This is true because third-degree block may progress to asystole and because the ventricular rate is usually very slow and ineffective. The heart rate of the ventricles may not be able to maintain a sufficient cardiac output needed to sustain life. Consequently, complete heart block is referred to as a lethal dysrhythmia.

In the truest sense of the term "complete," the atria and ventricles are completely blocked or separated from each other electrically. There is no communication between the atria and ventricles, as they literally beat independently of each other. The SA node fires at regular intervals, producing P waves at its normal rate of 60–100 beats per minute (bpm), whereas the ventricles are paced by an escape pacemaker in either the junctional tissues or the ventricles. If the ventricular pacemaker is the escape pacemaker, the ventricular rate will most commonly be between 20 and 40 bpm. If the resulting QRS complex is narrow, the escape pacemaker is located in the junctional tissue. If the QRS is widened, the escape pacemaker is located in the Purkinje network. There is, therefore, no relationship between the P waves and the QRS complexes.

The PR intervals will be variable in length. Some P waves may actually be "buried" inside the QRS complex and, therefore, not visible on the EKG strip. In this dysrhythmia, the "gate" actually closes and does not permit conduction of the initial electrical impulse through the AV junction or ventricles. This dysrhythmia is sometimes called *AV dissociation* because the atria and ventricles operate independently. This heart block may result from degenerative changes in the electrical conduction system (with advanced age), acute myocarditis, myocardial infarction, or drug toxicity.

As you carefully review Table 11–4 and the accompanying rhythm strips (Figure 11–4), you will recognize that the PR intervals are completely variable and that the P waves and QRS complexes have no relationship to each other. The pattern illustrates regularly occurring P waves and regularly occurring QRS complexes, but there is no ev-

Table 11–4

Third-degree (complete) heart block

Questions 1–5	Answers
1. What is the rate?	Atrial rate usually 60–100 bpm; ventricular rate based on site of escape pacemaker
2. What is the rhythm?	Atrial rhythm regular Ventricular rhythm regular
3. Is there a P wave before each QRS? Are the P waves upright and uniform?	No relationship to QRS complexes Yes
4. What is the length of the PR interval?	Totally variable; no pattern
5. Do all the QRS complexes look alike? What is the length of the QRS complexes?	Yes Based on site of escape pacemaker

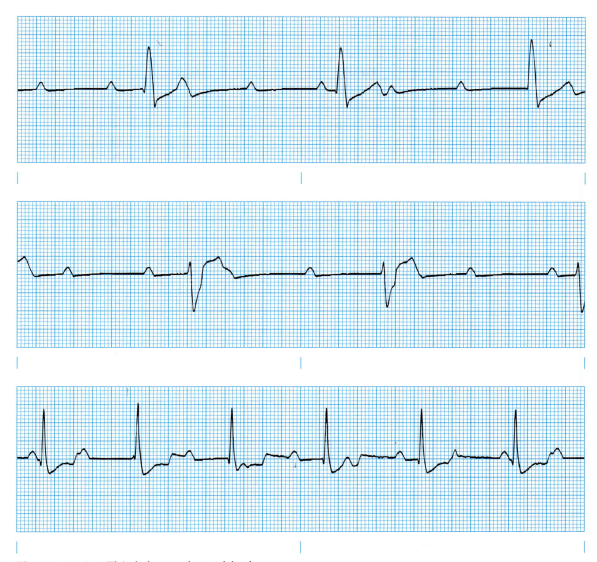

Figure 11–4.   Third-degree heart block

idence of a relationship between the two. In complete heart block, the R to R intervals should be constant.

Remember that complete heart block produces an EKG strip that shows no relationship between the P waves and QRS complexes; however, the atrial rate is regular, as is the ventricular rate. It is imperative that you observe the patient closely. **You must remember: Always monitor your patient's clinical condition!**

CLINICAL SIGNIFICANCE OF THE HEART BLOCK RHYTHMS

First-degree heart block

In and of itself, first-degree heart block is usually of little consequence. If this rhythm occurs in the face of an acute myocardial infarction, the patient must be closely observed and frequently assessed. Keep in mind, however, that this dysrhythmia may signal an initial progression to more advanced AV block.

Second-degree heart block, Mobitz type I (Wenckebach)

As stated earlier in this chapter, Mobitz type I is usually transient and often will revert to the patient's normal rhythm without outside intervention. If the EKG pattern demonstrates a rapid rate and frequently "dropped" beats, the patient's cardiac output may be compromised. Again, the importance of careful and diligent monitoring of the patient cannot be overemphasized. As with first-degree block, you must be alert to the possibility of advancing degrees of heart block.

Second-degree heart block, Mobitz type II

Mobitz II is the first of the more serious blocks that we have discussed in this chapter. It is prudent to remember that, often, Mobitz type II heart block will progress to third-degree heart block. The frequency of "dropped" beats (absences of QRS complexes) is a major concern in monitoring a patient who presents with this rhythm.

Recall that cardiac output may be seriously compromised. Be alert for signs and symptoms of decreased perfusion. These signs and symptoms may include syncope, decreased level of consciousness, angina, and other indications of hypoperfusion.

Third-degree (complete) heart block

Recall now that third-degree heart block is generally considered a lethal dysrhythmia, and act accordingly! The signs and symptoms exhibited by the patient who presents with third-degree block may be indicative of severe hypoperfusion; however, it is important to note that this is not **always** the case. Pay close attention to the width of the QRS complexes in order to determine whether the pacemaker site is ventricular or junctional.

By way of review, you should remember that the heart rate is based on the site of the pacemaker. If the QRS complexes are narrow and the patient is asymptomatic, the pacemaker cells in the AV junctional tissue are most likely serving as the pacemaker site. In this case the symptomatic patient may be treated with atropine, or pacing may be indicated. On the other hand, if the patient is exhibiting signs and symptoms and the QRS complexes are wide, transcutaneous pacing followed by the insertion of a transvenous pacemaker may be indicated.

Again, **listen to and observe** your patient, and never base your treatment decision on EKG strip analysis alone.

SUMMARY

Rhythms that are primarily disorders of conduction are called heart blocks. These rhythms occur when the electrical impulses that originate in the SA node are blocked or delayed in an area of the heart's electrical conduction system. Careful attention to, and evaluation of, the PR intervals is a critical component in the proper analysis of heart block rhythms.

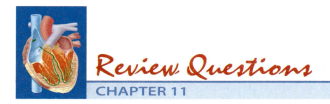

Review Questions
CHAPTER 11

1. When the EKG shows there is no relationship between the P wave and the QRS complex, you should suspect:

   a. First-degree block

   b. Second-degree block

   c. Third-degree block

   d. Electromechanical dissociation

2. Wenckebach differs from complete heart block in that CHB usually has a:

   a. Faster rate

   b. Normal QRS

   c. Constant PR interval

   d. Regular RR interval

3. PAT is a sudden onset of atrial tachycardia.

   a. True

   b. False

4. The keys to interpretation of second-degree heart block, Mobitz type II, are the presence of constant PR intervals and the fact that there are more P waves present than QRS complexes.

   a. True

   b. False

5. In order to calculate heart rate accurately by the R-to-R interval method, the patient must have a regular rhythm.

   a. True

   b. False

6. Proper application of EKG chest electrodes includes:

   a. Cleaning the patient's skin

   b. Drying the patient's skin

   c. Shaving the chest area of excess hair

   d. All of the above

7. It is prudent to remember that, often, Mobitz type II heart block will progress to third-degree heart block.

   a. True

   b. False

8. Typically, first degree block results from excessive conduction delay in the:

   a. SA node

   b. AV node

   c. Internodal pathways

   d. Purkinje network

9. Lead II is the lead most commonly used in the prehospital arena because it:

   a. Is easier to apply

   b. Shows good T waves

   c. Illustrates good P waves

   d. Is faster to apply

10. The heart block rhythm that most closely resembles a normal sinus rhythm is:

    a. Third-degree heart block

    b. Second-degree, Mobitz type I

    c. First-degree heart block

    d. Atrioventricular dissociation

11. It is important to note that the PR interval in Mobitz type II is constant, or regular, for every conducted beat.

    a. True

    b. False

12. The T wave on the EKG strip represents:

    a. Rest period

    b. Bundle of His

    c. Atrial contraction

    d. Ventricular contraction

13. If the ventricular pacemaker is the escape pacemaker, the ventricular rate will most commonly be between 20 and 40 bpm.

    a. True

    b. False

14. A prolonged PR interval is the hallmark of _____ degree block and is most commonly the only variation in the EKG strip.

    a. First-

    b. Third-

    c. Second-, type I

    d. Second-, type II

15. The first type of second-degree block is more serious than the second type because bradycardia is less likely to be present and because cardiac output is less likely to be seriously decreased in a second-degree type I block.

    a. True

    b. False

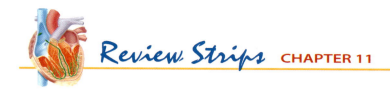

Review Strips   CHAPTER 11

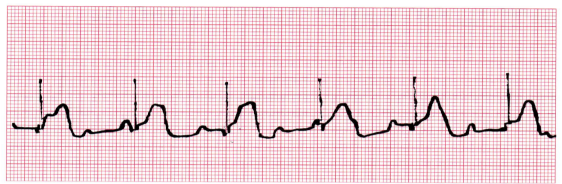

1. Rate _____   Rhythm _____

   P wave_____   PR interval_____

   QRS complex _____   Interpretation _____

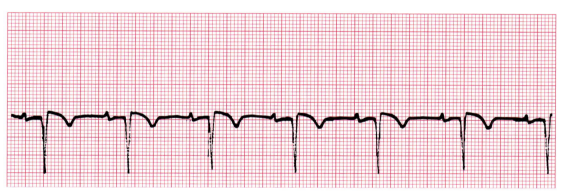

2. Rate _____   Rhythm _____

   P wave_____   PR interval_____

   QRS complex _____   Interpretation _____

8. Rate _____   Rhythm _____

   P wave_____   PR interval_____

   QRS complex _____   Iterpretation _____

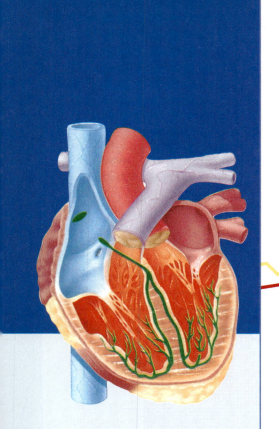

chapter 12

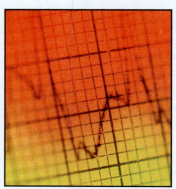

Introducing the Pacemaker Rhythms

objectives

Upon completion of this chapter, the student will be able to:

➤ Define the concept of an artificial pacemaker

➤ Describe transcutaneous pacing

➤ Discuss transvenous pacing

➤ List three types of permanent pacemakers

➤ Identify the indications for pacing

➤ Discuss the rules for interpretation of the pacemaker rhythms

➤ List common problems associated with pacemakers

➤ Explain the clinical significance of pacemaker rhythms

INTRODUCTION

An **artificial pacemaker** can be thought of as a device that substitutes for the normal pacemaker cells of the heart's electrical conduction system. An artificial pacemaker is, in the truest sense of the concept, an artificial regulator of heart rate. The use of artificial pacemakers may be necessitated when a patient's inherent electrical conduction pathway fails to function sufficiently. The EKG wave produced by an artificial pacemaker is referred to as a **pacemaker spike.**

Patients who experience signs and symptoms related to extensive disease of the sinus node (sick sinus syndrome), symptomatic bradycardia, or symptomatic complete heart block are often prime candidates for artificial pacing. Artificial pacemaker technology is advancing rapidly and is complex in nature. In this chapter, we will discuss some basic concepts regarding artificial pacemakers and the rhythms they produce. It is important for the health care professional to be able to recognize the presence of pacemaker rhythms on EKG strips in order to make prudent decisions about treatment.

Whether temporary or permanent, artificial pacemakers are small devices that initiate electrical impulses in specific locations in the myocardial tissue. Artificial pacemakers have two basic parts: the generator and the lead wires. The **generator** controls the rate and strength of each electrical impulse. The **lead wires** have an electrode at the tip and relay the electrical impulse from the generator to the myocardium.

Temporary pacemakers are used to sustain a patient's heart rate in emergent situations, whereas **permanent pacemakers** are implanted inside the patient's upper left chest (most commonly) and are left in place. The following discussion provides an overview of common considerations regarding artificial pacemakers.

TEMPORARY PACING

Transcutaneous pacing

Transcutaneous pacing, often abbreviated **TCP,** is also commonly called external cardiac pacing. Initially introduced in the early 1950s, TCP was used to treat serious symptoms associated with complete heart block. The device quickly fell out of favor, primarily because of its marked disadvantages, such as patients' complaints of associated pain and EKG aberrations secondary to muscle contractions. Only in the past 20 years have modern technological advances made TCP an acceptable and often effective modality for rhythms such as symptomatic bradycardia, symptomatic complete heart block, and other rhythm disturbances.

The American Heart Association (AHA) has now recognized and recommended the use of transcutaneous pacemaker devices in both the bradycardia and the asystole algorithms. Because TCP can be initiated quickly and is not as invasive as other pacing methods, the AHA has recommended it as the suggested treatment of choice in emergent cardiac care settings.

Transcutaneous pacing consists of two large electrode pads, which are most commonly placed in an anterior-posterior position on the patient's chest to conduct electrical

artificial pacemaker a device that substitutes for the normal pacemaker cells of the heart's electrical conduction system

pacemaker spike the EKG wave produced by an artificial pacemaker

generator controls the rate and strength of each electrical impulse

lead wires relay the electrical impulse from the generator to the myocardium

temporary pacemakers used to sustain a patient's heart rate in emergent situations

permanent pacemakers implanted inside the patient's upper left chest (most commonly) and are left in place

transcutaneous pacing (TCP), commonly called external cardiac pacing, consists of two large electrode pads, which are most commonly placed in an anterior-posterior position on the patient's chest to conduct electrical impulses through the skin to the heart impulses through the skin to the heart. Utilizing this method, the cardiac muscle cells depolarize in a normal fashion.

Before the implementation of TCP, the patient should be placed in a supine position, and an IV, oxygen, and EKG monitoring must be established. Most prehospital care systems require that the prehospital provider receive orders from medical control prior to initiating TCP.

Symptomatic bradycardia or asystole must be confirmed prior to implementing TCP procedures. After the electrode pads and the electrodes are properly placed, the desired heart rate should be set. This rate is commonly in the range of 60–80 beats per minute (bpm). The initial voltage setting is at 0 amperes before the pacer is turned on.

capture noted by the presence of a spike and wide QRS complexes, the presence of an adequate carotid pulse and blood pressure, and an increased level of consciousness

Although recommendations vary regarding initial current settings, it is universally agreed that the ampere setting be **gradually** increased until capture is accomplished. **Capture** is usually noted by the presence of a spike and wide QRS complexes, the presence of an adequate carotid pulse and blood pressure, and an increased level of consciousness. The prehospital provider must be in voice contact with medical control, and the patient's overall clinical condition must be constantly monitored. Keep in mind that the preset heart rate and the amperage may need to be adjusted because of various factors such as the patient's movement or changes in the patient's underlying heart rhythm. Rhythm strips should be gathered, and concise, detailed documentation is required. At times, the patient may experience mild discomfort secondary to TCP implementation. If pain or discomfort is evident, the medical control or the attending physician should be notified. He or she will, in most instances, order sedation to be administered to the patient.

Transvenous pacing

transvenous pacing (through a vein) a lead wire is inserted through the skin and threaded into a large vein leading into the right side of the heart and controlled by an external power source

Transvenous (through a vein) pacing is another method for delivering electrical impulses to the myocardial tissue. In transvenous pacing, a lead wire is inserted through the skin and threaded into a large vein leading into the right side of the heart and controlled by an external power source. The electrical impulses generated by the external power source stimulate the right atrium or the right ventricle and travel through the electrical conduction system, producing depolarization. Note that transvenous pacing is more invasive in nature than TCP, due to the necessity of venipuncture for the purpose of inserting the lead wire.

fixed-rate or asynchronous pacemaker programmed to deliver electrical impulses at a constant selected rate

Pacemakers are preset, or programmed, to pace (or deliver electrical impulses) in two modes. A **fixed-rate** or **asynchronous pacemaker** is programmed to deliver electrical impulses at a constant selected rate. A **demand** or **synchronous pacemaker** generates electrical impulses when the patient's heart rate falls below a predetermined rate. Fixed-rate pacemakers are not commonly used in today's advanced technology.

PERMANENT PACING

demand or synchronous pacemaker generates electrical impulses when the patient's heart rate falls below a predetermined rate

Permanent, or implanted, pacemakers are most commonly used when patients present with signs of symptomatic bradycardia or complete heart block that have not responded to pharmacologic interventions. As stated earlier in this chapter, a permanent pacemaker consists of a surgically implanted generator and a lead wire that is introduced into the heart through a central vein.

The three primary types of permanent pacemakers used today are the atrial, ventricular, and AV sequential pacemakers. Descriptions of these three types follow.

a. ***Atrial pacemakers.*** – The lead wire electrode is inserted into the right atrium. The pacemaker's electrical impulse first stimulates the atrium and then travels down the electrical conduction pathway through the ventricles (Figure 12–1).

b. ***Ventricular pacemakers.*** – The lead wire electrode is inserted into the right ventricle. The electrical impulse from the pacemaker generator produces ventricular depolarization (Figure 12–2).

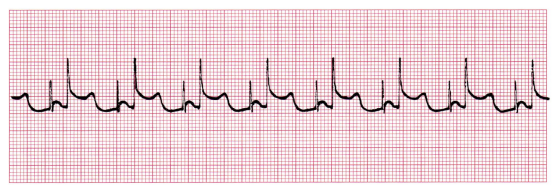

Figure 12–1.   Atrial pacemaker

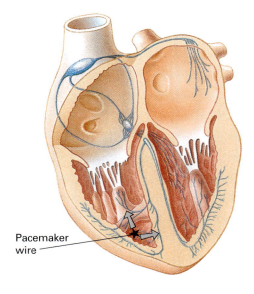

Pacemaker wire

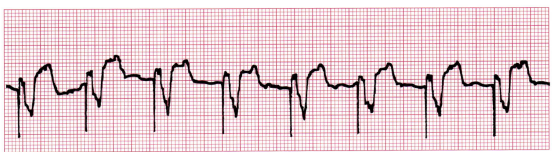

Figure 12–2.   Ventricular pacemaker

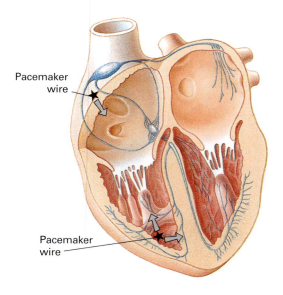

Pacemaker
wire

Pacemaker
wire

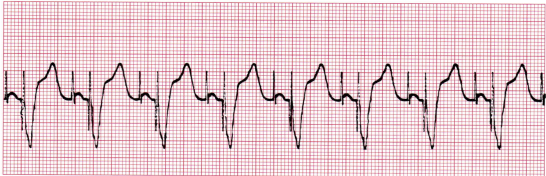

Figure 12–3. Atrioventricular sequential pacemaker

c. *AV sequential pacemakers.* – This is the most commonly used type of permanent pacemaker. There are two electrodes on the lead wire: one is placed in the right atrium and one is placed in the right ventricle. Artificial impulses stimulate, or pace, first the atria, then the ventricles (Figure 12–3).

INDICATIONS FOR PACING

Artificial pacemakers may be indicated for patients who present with persistent and symptomatic second-degree type II heart block, complete heart block, occurrences of severe symptomatic bradycardia, or sick sinus syndrome. Transcutaneous pacing may be used as a temporary bridge modality in severe, symptomatic bradycardia-related rhythms, until transvenous pacing or permanent pacing can be established. Transcutaneous pacing may also be used in cardiac arrest or profound bradycardia, secondary to drug overdose, or in the rare event of failure of a permanent pacemaker.

RULES FOR INTERPRETATION OF PACEMAKER RHYTHMS

While analyzing an EKG strip produced by an artificial pacemaker, you should apply the five-step approach, just as you have done with the dysrhythmias in the previous chapters of this text. Consider Table 12–1 and Figure 12–4.

Table 12–1

Artificial pacemaker rhythm

Questions 1–5	Answers
1. What is the rate?	Varies according to preset rate of pacemaker
2. What is the rhythm?	Regular if pacing is fixed; irregular if demand-paced
3. Is there a P wave before each QRS? Are the P waves upright and uniform?	May be absent or present, depending on type of artificial pacemaker
4. What is the length of the PR interval?	Variable, depending on type of artificial pacemaker
5. Do all the QRS complexes look alike? What is the length of the QRS complexes?	Usually; greater than 0.12 second; bizarre morphology; presence of spikes

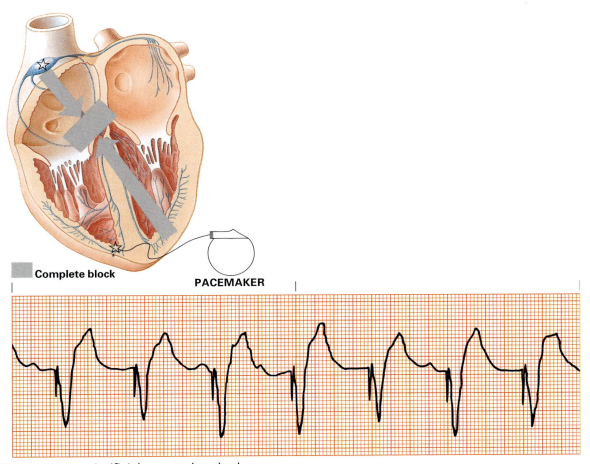

■ **Complete block**   **PACEMAKER**

Figure 12–4.   Artificial pacemaker rhythm

Remember that properly functioning pacemakers will produce rhythms with pacemaker spikes. The pacemaker spikes are usually readily identifiable; however, some of the newer cardiac monitors do not pick up the pacemaker spike on either the oscilloscope or the graph paper. It is essential that you realize that the presence of pacemaker spikes indicates only that the pacemaker is firing; pacemaker spikes do not reveal information relative to ventricular contraction. Assess your patient for the presence of symptoms. **Remember: Always monitor your patient's clinical condition!**

COMMON PROBLEMS ASSOCIATED WITH PACEMAKERS

Battery failure

Decreased amplitude of the pacemaker spike and a slowing pacemaker rate may both be caused by battery failure. Most pacemaker batteries are based on today's modern technology and have long lives. Periodic pacemaker battery checks are usually made by the patient's physician, preventing the occurrence of battery failure. In the unlikely event of complete battery failure, the pacemaker will fail to function and the patient's underlying rhythm may return or cardiac arrest may result. Depending on the underlying rhythm and patient's symptoms, battery failure can be considered a dire emergency.

Runaway pacemakers

Fortunately, situations in which a pacemaker rhythm "runs away" are rarely seen today, especially with newer pacemakers. However, when this problem is identified, a rapid rate of electrical impulse discharge results. At times, the discharge rate may reach 200–300 beats per minute. Today's newer generators provide a gradual increase in rate as their battery currents decrease. Management of patients who exhibit evidence of runaway pacemaker rhythms consists of immediate transport to a definitive care facility.

Failure to capture

When an artificial pacemaker successfully depolarizes the specified chamber or chambers of the heart, as denoted by the presence of a pacemaker spike followed by a P wave or QRS complex, capture has occurred.

When lead wires become displaced or a pacemaker battery fails, the pacemaker can fail to capture. When failure to capture occurs, pacemaker spikes will be visible on the EKG strip, but you will note that the pacer spikes are not followed by a QRS complex. Common causes of failure to capture include displacement of lead wire electrodes and battery failure.

sensing is simply the capability of a pacemaker to recognize inherent electrical conduction system activity

Failure of sensing devices in demand pacemakers

Demand pacemakers contain a sensing device. **Sensing** is simply the capability of a pacemaker to recognize inherent electrical activity. If a patient spontaneously develops an adequate heart rate, the demand pacemaker may fail to shut down. If this occurs, the heart's normal heart rate may compete with the rate of the demand pace-maker. In this event, the pacemaker may fire at an inopportune time, such as the vul-nerable or relative refractory period during ventricular repolarization, and ventricular fibrillation may ensue. This situation is a dire emergency and must be treated accordingly.

The pacemaker may fail to sense as a result of displacement of the electrode tip, battery failure, lead wire breakage, or significant metabolic variants. Management of a pacemaker that has failed to sense includes correcting the underlying problem.

CLINICAL SIGNIFICANCE OF PACEMAKER RHYTHMS

Under normal circumstances, patients with artificial pacemakers require no unique medical attention. It is critical to note, however, that pacemaker failure produces a life-threatening event in patients whose underlying rhythm is insufficient to maintain cardiac output and adequate systemic perfusion. In these situations, the patient should be immediately trans-ported to a definitive care facility for further intervention.

The vast majority of today's modern artificial pacemakers present no problems. In fact, some of today's pacemakers have dual functions in that they not only are capable of pacing the heart but also recognize certain dysrhythmias and defibrillate, if indicated.

It is also important to note that problems with pacemakers usually occur within the first month after implantation. Occasional problems associated with the implantation procedure may include pneumothorax, induced cardiac dysrhythmias, bleeding, and very rarely air embolus.

Whenever you encounter an unconscious patient, you should remember to exam-ine the patient for the presence of a medic alert apparatus, as well as for a small palpa-ble mass underneath the skin in the patient's upper chest or upper abdomen. The presence of either may alert you to the probability of an implanted artificial pacemaker.

Dysrhythmias associated with pacemaker failure are treated the same as dysrhyth-mias in any other patient. Although patients with pacemakers should be defibrillated like other patients, it is important to note that the defibrillator paddles should not be dis-charged directly over the battery pack.

SUMMARY

Artificial pacemakers have the capability to produce an electrical stimulus when the heart's inherent electrical conduction ability is compromised. This is accomplished through the implantation of electrodes within the heart. These artificial pacemakers are classified as transcutaneous, transvenous, or permanent. Medical science has advanced to the point where problems with pacemakers are rare.

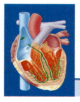

Review Questions
CHAPTER 12

1. AV sequential pacemakers stimulate only the atria.
   a. False
   b. True

2. _____ is indicated on an EKG strip when there is a P wave or QRS complex following each pacemaker spike.
   a. Sensing
   b. Capture
   c. Loss of sensing
   d. Loss of capture

3. Atrial pacemakers are commonly used today.
   a. True
   b. False

4. The two types of temporary pacemakers include the transvenous pacemaker and the _____ pacemaker.
   a. Ventricular
   b. Atrial
   c. Transcutaneous
   d. Sensing

5. Indications for the use of artificial pacemakers include:
   a. Asymptomatic bradycardia
   b. Symptomatic complete heart block
   c. Asymptomatic second-degree heart block
   d. First-degree heart block

6. The EKG wave produced by an artificial pacemaker is referred to as a (an):
   a. Pacemaker spike
   b. Ectopic focus
   c. Aberration
   d. Anomaly

7. The American Heart Association (AHA) has now recognized the use of transcutaneous pacemaker devices in both the bradycardia and the asystole algorithms.
   a. True
   b. False

8. Ventricular asystole represents an absence of all ventricular electrical activity on an EKG strip.

    a. True

    b. False

9. Symptomatic bradycardia must be confirmed prior to implementing TCP procedures.

    a. False

    b. True

10. Possible problems associated with pacemakers include:

    a. Battery failure

    b. Failure to capture

    c. Failure to sense

    d. All of the above

11. Transvenous (through a vein) pacing is another method for delivering electrical impulses to the myocardial tissue.

    a. True

    b. False

12. TCP consists of two large electrode pads, which are most commonly placed in an anterior-posterior position on the patient's chest in order to conduct electrical impulses through the skin to the heart.

    a. True

    b. False

13. Under normal circumstances, patients with artificial pacemakers require no unique medical attention.

    a. True

    b. False

14. Dysrhythmias associated with pacemaker failure are treated the same as dysrhythmias in any other patient.

    a. True

    b. False

15. Although patients with pacemakers should be defibrillated like any other patient, it is important to note that the defibrillator paddles should not be discharged directly over the battery pack.

    a. True

    b. False

Review Strips CHAPTER 12

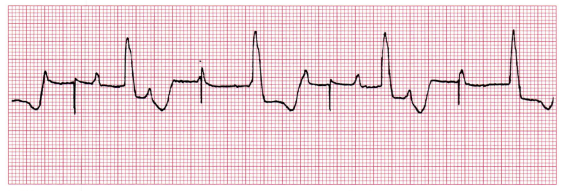

1. Rate _____   Rhythm _____

   P wave_____   PR interval_____

   QRS complex _____   Interpretation _____

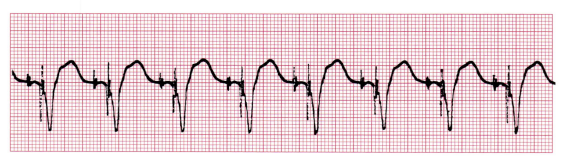

2. Rate _____   Rhythm _____

   P wave_____   PR interval_____

   QRS complex _____   Interpretation _____

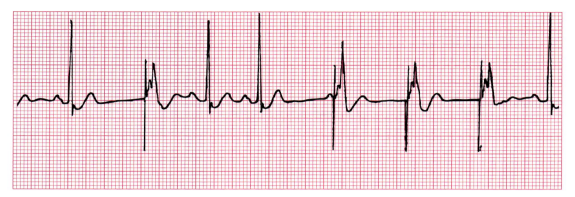

3. Rate _____ Rhythm _____
   P wave_____ PR interval_____
   QRS complex _____ Interpretation _____

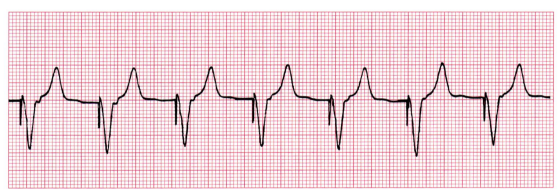

4. Rate _____ Rhythm _____
   P wave_____ PR interval_____
   QRS complex _____ Interpretation _____

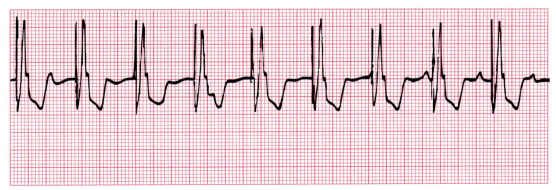

5. Rate _____ Rhythm _____
   P wave_____ PR interval_____
   QRS complex _____ Interpretation _____

INTRODUCTION

Cardiac emergencies, including acute myocardial infarction (AMI), continue to be one of the nation's leading causes of death. Heart attacks and other cardiac emergencies affect more than five million individuals each year. More than one million deaths each year are directly attributed to heart disease. Your thorough understanding of the clinical picture of patients who present with cardiac emergencies will enhance your ability to assess and treat these patients in a more time-efficient manner.

CHEST PAIN

Cardiac versus noncardiac

Chest pain of cardiac origin may present in various ways. This type of chest pain may be indicative of serious illness, myocardial ischemia, myocardial injury, or simply stress or exercise-related hypoxia.

chest pain is the most common presenting symptom of cardiac disease, as well as the most common complaint by patients

Chest pain is the most common presenting symptom of cardiac disease, as well as the most common complaint by patients. Chest pain of cardiac origin is typically described as "crushing" or "squeezing" in nature and is commonly associated with nausea, vomiting, and **diaphoresis** (profuse sweating). The pain is often located substernally and may radiate to the jaw, shoulder, arm, and one or more fingers, most commonly on the left side (Figure 13–1).

diaphoresis profuse sweating

Chest pain from an acute myocardial infarction may escalate in intensity. Patients may express a feeling of "impending doom" and may exhibit extreme anxiety. A common obstacle to timely intervention by a health care provider dealing with a patient who complains of chest pain is denial. Patients often deny the possibility that they may indeed be experiencing a heart attack, thinking, "It can't happen to me."

Often patients prefer to believe that they are merely experiencing "indigestion" and that the symptoms will be gone by morning. Unfortunately, it may be the patient rather than the symptoms who is gone by morning. However, with proper public education many lives have been saved that otherwise would have been lost; this is due in large part to the simple fact that many hundreds of laypersons have been certified in the skill of cardiopulmonary resuscitation (CPR).

neuropathy inability to perceive pain due to diseases of the nerves

It should be noted that in special circumstances patients may experience no chest pain at all and may still have sustained a myocardial infarction. This is true primarily in the diabetic patient with advanced **neuropathy** due to destruction of nerve endings, causing an inability to perceive pain due to diseases of the nerves. The scenario with which diabetic patients may present is often with congestive heart failure. Some elderly patients may experience an AMI without chest pain; most commonly their only presenting symptom will be a complaint of profound weakness.

Noncardiac causes of chest pain

Causes of noncardiac chest pain are numerous. However, you should remember that chest pain is cardiac in nature until proved otherwise, especially in the prehospital arena.

Causes of noncardiac chest pain include (but are not limited to) the following:

Pleurisy—inflammation of the covering of the lungs (pleura)
Costrochondritis—inflammation of intercostal muscles (located between ribs)

EARLY SIGNS OF HEART ATTACK

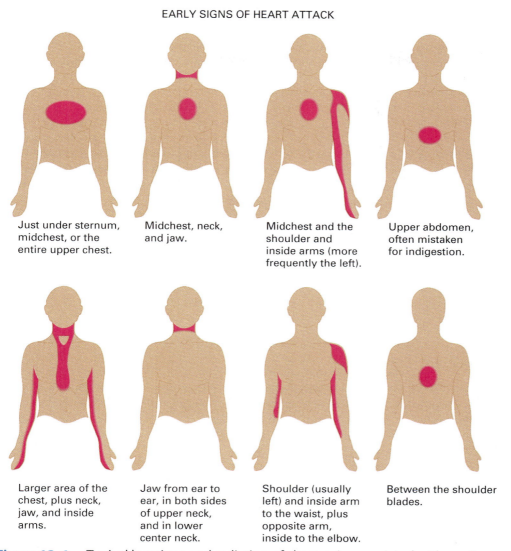

Just under sternum, midchest, or the entire upper chest.

Midchest, neck, and jaw.

Midchest and the shoulder and inside arms (more frequently the left).

Upper abdomen, often mistaken for indigestion.

Larger area of the chest, plus neck, jaw, and inside arms.

Jaw from ear to ear, in both sides of upper neck, and in lower center neck.

Shoulder (usually left) and inside arm to the waist, plus opposite arm, inside to the elbow.

Between the shoulder blades.

Figure 13–1.   Typical locations and radiation of chest pain associated with cardiac emergencies

Pericarditis—inflammation of the pericardial sac (surrounding the heart)
Myocardial contusion—secondary to chest trauma (high incidence of dysrhythmias)
Muscle strain—secondary to overstretching of the chest wall muscles
Trauma—secondary to an injury to the chest wall or to organs contained within the chest (or both)

Examples of chest injuries secondary to trauma include:

Hemothorax—collection of blood within the pleural cavity
Pneumothorax—the collection of air within the pleural cavity
Hemopneumothorax—collection of blood and air within the pleural cavity
Tension pneumothorax—air trapped in the thoracic cavity without an escape route; pressure builds and affects the lungs, heart, and other vital organs

angina pectoris
pain that results from a reduction in blood supply to myocardial tissue

atherosclerosis
narrowed coronary arterial walls, secondary to fatty deposits

"stable" or predictable angina a particular activity may elicit chest pain

unstable angina
pain not elicited by activity that most commonly occurs while the patient is at rest; also referred to as "preinfarctional" angina

Prinzmetal's angina or vasospastic angina form of angina that can occur when the coronary arteries experience spasms and constrict

Chest trauma can produce severe chest pain and may indicate a serious condition that requires immediate intervention. Any patient who exhibits chest pain, regardless of the clinical presentation, should be monitored for possible dysrhythmias. Remember the old adage, "An ounce of prevention. . . ." when dealing with chest pain. This adage applies because TIME IS MUSCLE!

ANGINA PECTORIS

Angina pectoris is pain that results from a reduction in blood supply to myocardial tissue. The pain is typically temporary. If blood flow is quickly restored, little or no permanent change or damage may result. Angina is characterized by chest pain or discomfort deep in the sternal area and is often described as heaviness, pressure, or moderately severe pain. It is quite often mistaken for indigestion. This pain can be referred to the neck, lower jaw, left shoulder, arm, and fingers.

Angina pectoris most often results from narrowed or hardened coronary arterial walls (Figure 13–2), commonly caused by **atherosclerosis.** This reduction in blood flow results in a reduced supply of oxygen to cardiac muscle cells.

The pain is often predictably associated with exercise and is due to the increased pumping activity of the heart, which then requires more oxygen that the narrowed blood vessels cannot supply. This may be referred to as **"stable"** or **predictable angina,** in that a particular activity may elicit chest pain. The symptoms of stable angina will usually respond well to appropriate treatment, including rest and the administration of oxygen.

Conversely, the pain of **unstable angina** is not elicited by activity and most commonly occurs while the patient is at rest. It is not unusual for these patients to report to you that they were awakened from sleep as a result of significant chest pain. Unstable angina generally indicates a progression of atherosclerotic heart disease and is also referred to as "preinfarctional" angina.

Yet another form of angina can occur when the coronary arteries experience spasms and constrict, thus significantly decreasing myocardial oxygenation. This type of angina is commonly referred to as **Prinzmetal's angina** or **vasospastic angina.** It is

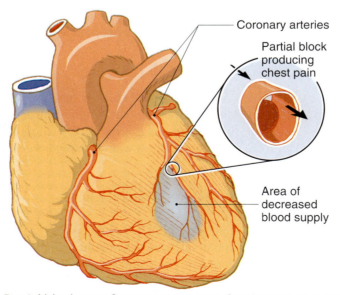

Coronary arteries

Partial block producing chest pain

Area of decreased blood supply

Figure 13–2.   Partial blockage of a coronary artery deprives an area in the myocardium of oxygen and results in chest pain, or angina pectoris

interesting to note that, in some cases, when a 12-lead EKG is obtained from a patient who is experiencing Prinzmetal's angina, there may be evidence of EKG changes consistent with myocardial injury. However, a 12-lead EKG obtained after nitroglycerin has been administered may illustrate no pattern of injury. In this event, the vasodilation produced by the nitroglycerin alleviated the myocardial ischemia that led to the abnormal EKG. It may be significant to note that while the majority of patients who experience Prinzmetal's angina have underlying atherosclerotic disease, some may have little or none.

Management of the patient who is experiencing angina should center on decreasing the workload of the heart. There are many ways to accomplish this objective, including these:

➤ Place the patient at rest, in a calm, quiet environment.
➤ Provide appropriate reassurance to the patient.
➤ Obtain a 12-lead EKG, if possible.
➤ Administer oxygen at a high flow rate in order to increase myocardial oxygenation.
➤ Establish IV line to ensure that a lifeline for administration of fluid is available.
➤ Administer nitroglycerin (per medical direction).

Nitroglycerin causes dilation of the blood vessels that consequently reduces the workload of the heart—thus reducing the need for oxygen because the heart has to pump blood against a lesser pressure. The blood tends to remain in the dilated blood vessels, and less blood is returned to the heart for distribution.

An important tool in the diligent management of patients who experience chest pain centers on the necessity of follow-up evaluation. Oftentimes, when the pain goes away, the patient tends to forget that it occurred. Hence, the healthcare provider must assume the role of patient educator in order to emphasize the importance of further evaluation. Let's face it . . . if a patient experiences enough pain to cause an ambulance to be summoned or causing a trip to the Emergency Department to occur, it stands to reason that this pain needs to be evaluated. We must be diligent and patient, but persistent and persuasive in these efforts.

A complaint of chest pain should never be minimized. All patients who experience chest pain should be strongly encouraged to be evaluated by a physician. As health care providers we should remember that denial continues to be an obstacle in the care and management of some patients who experience chest pain.

ACUTE MYOCARDIAL INFARCTION

An **acute myocardial infarction** results from a prolonged lack of blood flow to a portion of the myocardial tissue and results in a lack of oxygen. Eventually, myocardial cellular death will follow. Myocardial infarctions vary with the amount of myocardial tissue and the portion of the heart affected. If blood supply to cardiac muscle is reestablished within 10–20 minutes, there will usually be no permanent injury. If oxygen deprivation lasts longer, cellular death will result. Within 30 to 60 seconds after blockage of a coronary blood vessel, functional changes will become evident. The electrical properties of the cardiac muscle will be altered, and the ability of the cardiac muscle to function properly is lost.

The most common cause of myocardial infarction is **thrombus formation** that blocks a coronary artery (Figure 13–3). Coronary arteries narrowed by atherosclerotic damage are one of the conditions that increase the likelihood of myocardial infarction.

nitroglycerin
causes dilation of the blood vessels that consequently reduces the workload of the heart

acute myocardial infarction (heart attack)
results from a prolonged lack of blood flow to a portion of the myocardial tissue and results in a lack of oxygen

thrombus formation the most common cause of myocardial infarction, results in blockage of the coronary artery

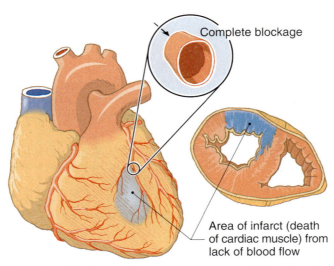

Figure 13–3.   Complete blockage of a coronary artery will lead to the death of myocardium due to lack of oxygen, and to a resulting myocardial infarction

Atherosclerotic lesions partially block blood vessels, resulting in disorderly blood flow, as the surfaces of the lesions are rough. These changes increase the probability of thrombus formation.

Patient assessment and management

In order to assess the patient with chest pain properly, you must be able to recognize the common signs and symptoms. Signs and symptoms of an acute myocardial infarction may be quite similar to those of angina pectoris. Clear differences include the fact that the pain caused by an AMI lasts longer and is usually not relieved by rest (Table 13–1).

The goal of management of the patient with symptomatic chest pain is to interrupt the infarction process. This can be achieved through interventions such as immediate and effective administration of oxygen, alleviation of pain, management of dysrhythmias, and possibly initiation of thrombolytic therapy in order to limit the progression of the infarct.

It is imperative to learn and remember that "time is muscle" and act accordingly. Thus timely assessment and management, including immediate administration of oxygen, must be rapidly initiated and completed within a 10-minute interval. Your initial assessment and evaluation should focus on the patient's general appearance. You will probably note that patients who are suffering from an AMI will tend to remain quiet and still. These patients also tend to prefer a sitting position. The Fowler's or semi-Fowler's position tends to allow the patient to breathe more comfortably and may decrease the workload of the myocardium.

A thorough and timely evaluation and management of the patient's ABCs is imperative. Any problem encountered during this evaluation must be managed quickly and must be followed by a rapid assessment of the vital signs. Because of the wide variations of the presenting vital signs, the clinician should be aware that vital signs are not necessarily reliable in diagnosing an AMI. In spite of this fact, it is important that you monitor and record these signs at frequent intervals.

One of the most important assessment tools that you will use when managing a suspected AMI patient is the cardiac monitor. Dysrhythmias that originate from ischemic and injured myocardial tissues are a common complication of acute myocardial infarctions.

Table 13–1

Differential symptomology: AMI versus angina	
Signs and Symptoms— Angina Pectoris	**Signs and Symptoms— Acute Myocardial Infarction**
Chest pain: short duration, usually lasts 3–10 minutes, usually relieved by nitroglycerin	Chest pain: usually lasts more than 2 hours; not relieved by nitroglycerin
Brought on by stress or exercise and relieved by rest	Usually not precipitated by exercise or stress; not relieved by rest
May be accompanied by dysrhythmias	Usually accompanied by dysrhythmias
Patients usually do not experience nausea, vomiting, or diaphoresis	Patients will commonly complain of nausea and vomiting and are often profoundly diaphoretic

It is critical to understand that in the clinical setting, dysrhythmias may be simply warning signs or may signal severe life-threatening events. In either case, you must not ignore the presence of any abnormal heart rhythm when dealing with a patient who exhibits a "textbook" clinical presentation of an acute myocardial infarction. Although the three-lead EKG strip will depict the heart rate and rhythm adequately, the 12-lead EKG has the ability to afford a comprehensive picture of the myocardial events occurring during an acute myocardial infarction. For an in-depth discussion relative to 12-lead EKGs, please refer to this book's companion text, *Understanding 12-Lead EKGs: A Practical Approach.*

Your suspicion of an acute myocardial infarction must be based on the combination of a positive 12-lead EKG and the patient's clinical "picture" (signs and symptoms), in the prehospital arena. Keep in mind that a negative 12-lead EKG does *NOT* rule out the presence of an AMI. Remember also that any patients who complain of chest pain must be thoroughly evaluated, and their management should continue until the possibility of AMI is ruled out by the physician.

Without a doubt, the most important drug that any patient with chest pain can receive is **oxygen.** Time and again, in this and other textbooks, you will see that statement— simply because it is true and it is critically important to the viability of your patient.

Other considerations regarding treatment include:

➤ 100 percent oxygen
➤ Establish an IV lifeline (according to local protocols)
➤ Measure oxygen saturation level (pulse oximetry), if equipment is available
➤ Continuous cardiac monitoring
➤ Pain control and management—nitroglycerin, morphine sulfate, demerol, etc. (according to local protocols)
➤ Thrombolytic therapy, aspirin

Remember that the focus of assessment and treatment of the patient who presents with chest pain centers on the immediate oxygenation of hypoxic tissue. Treatment initiatives will vary, depending upon your patient's specific situation; however, you must focus on continual and thorough assessment until such time as the patient is clinically stable.

As mentioned at the beginning of this chapter, cardiac emergencies, including acute myocardial infarction, continue to be one of the nation's leading causes of death. Thus the significance of the patient's condition, as well as the need for early intervention for

oxygen the most important drug that any patient with chest pain can receive

a patient with suspected AMI, is paramount. An acute myocardial infarction may be a staggering event involving disturbances of the electrical conduction system as well as mechanical failure secondary to infarcted tissue.

HEART FAILURE

heart failure the inability of the myocardium to meet the cardiac output demands of the body

For many years, the term "heart failure" was considered by many to refer to a singular disease process, divided subsequently into simply left or right heart failure. In more recent years, heart failure, along with all its variations, has been more correctly regarded as a clinical syndrome. **Heart failure** can be simply defined as the inability of the myocardium to meet the cardiac output demands of the body.

Heart failure may occur from a variety of determinants, including, but not limited to, the following:

➤ Coronary disease
➤ Valvular disease
➤ Myocardial injury

Other clinical symptomologies that may influence heart disease include:

➤ Dysrhythmias
➤ Hypertension
➤ Pulmonary emboli
➤ Systemic sepsis
➤ Electrolyte disturbances

Left ventricular failure

left ventricular failure when a patient's left ventricle ceases to function in an adequate capacity as to sustain sufficient systemic cardiac output

When a patient's left ventricle ceases to function in an adequately capacity as to sustain sufficient systemic cardiac output, regardless of the specific cause, this condition is referred to as **left ventricular failure.** In considering the physiology of left heart failure, it is important to recall that blood has been delivered appropriately into the cavity; however, the myocardial musculature of the left ventricle cannot contract sufficiently to empty the blood into the systemic circulation.

As a result of the insufficient emptying of the left ventricle, stroke volume is decreased. When stroke volume is decreased, the body's compensatory mechanisms (increased heart rate, vasoconstriction, etc.) begin to function at an accelerated rate, in an effort to restore organ perfusion. As a consequence of these mechanisms, pressure in the right as well as the left atrium rises dramatically. It is at this point that the overloaded heart pushes the blood back into the pulmonary system. This backup in the pulmonary system causes plasma to mix with and displace alveolar air, resulting in **pulmonary edema.** This influx of fluid into the alveoli impedes the ability of the alveoli to function properly; thus gas exchange is severely compromised. This compromise, if not correctly promptly, eventually leads to **hypoxia.**

pulmonary edema backup of blood in the pulmonary system that causes plasma to mix with and displace alveolar air

Due to the engorgement of the alveoli, the patient may present with the characteristic symptom of pink, frothy sputum and significant dyspnea. It is important to remember that if left untreated, severe left heart failure can lead to extreme hypoxia and subsequent death.

hypoxia low oxygen level

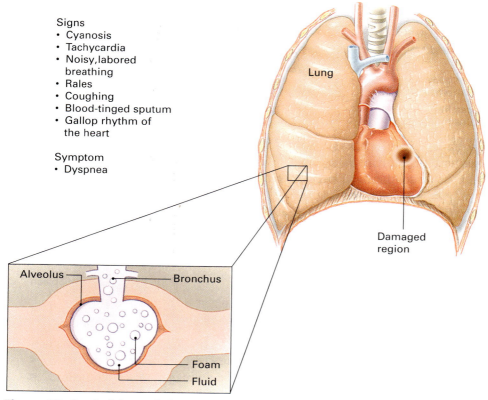

LEFT HEART FAILURE

Signs
• Cyanosis
• Tachycardia
• Noisy, labored
  breathing
• Rales
• Coughing
• Blood-tinged sputum
• Gallop rhythm of
  the heart

Symptom
• Dyspnea

Lung

Damaged
region

Alveolus

Bronchus

Foam

Fluid

Figure 13–4. Left heart failure

Emergency management of left heart failure (Figure 13–4) is aimed at decreasing myocardial oxygen demand, improving myocardial contractility, and improving oxygenation and ventilation. Factors to consider in the treatment and management of left heart failure include these:

➤ Allow the patient to assume a position of comfort; if clinically feasible, the patient's legs should be allowed to dangle off the bed or cot.
➤ Provide 100 percent high-flow oxygenation via a nonrebreather mask.
➤ Utilize pulse oximetry to maintain O_2 saturation of at least 95 percent.
➤ Carefully monitor the patient's LOC for signs of deterioration.
➤ Establish IV line at KVO (keep vein open) rate; carefully restrict intake.
➤ Establish and maintain EKG monitoring and obtain EKG strip.
➤ Obtain permission from medical control physician, or follow local protocol for administration of medication (or both).

Medications commonly prescribed to treat the patient experiencing left heart failure include:

➤ Morphine sulfate
➤ Furosemide (Lasix)
➤ Nitroglycerin

RIGHT HEART FAILURE

➤ Hypotension (may be extreme)
➤ Dyspnea
➤ Weak, rapid pulse

Beck's triad
muffled heart sounds, JVD, and narrowing pulse pressure

pulsus paradoxus
evidenced by a systolic blood pressure that drops more than 10–15 mmHg during inspiration

Sometimes referred to as **"Beck's triad,"** muffled heart sounds, JVD, and narrowing pulse pressure are commonly called the "classic" indicators of cardiac tamponade. A **pulsus paradoxus,** as evidenced by a systolic blood pressure that drops more than 10–15 mmHg during inspiration, may also occur with cardiac tamponade.

Emergency management of cardiac tamponade includes the following:

➤ Ensure and maintain a patent airway.
➤ Administer 100 percent high-flow oxygen.
➤ Monitor pulse oximetry—maintain O_2 saturation of 95 percent.
➤ Establish and maintain IV support.
➤ Administer pharmacological agents as indicated.
➤ Transport expeditiously.

The therapy of choice involves intervention by the physician, in most instances. Called a pericardiocentesis, this invasive procedure consists of aspiration of fluid from the pericardium with a needle. Remember, cardiac tamponade is a true medical emergency. If the patient is to survive this dire condition, the pericardial blood must be removed and the source of bleeding stopped.

CARDIOGENIC SHOCK

cardiogenic shock when left ventricular function is so severely compromised that the heart can no longer meet the metabolic requirements of the body

hypovolemia
decreased blood volume

When left ventricular function is so severely compromised that the heart can no longer meet the metabolic requirements of the body, **cardiogenic shock** may occur. This condition is often a result of extensive myocardial infarction and is said to be the most critical form of heart failure. Ineffective myocardial contractions result in a marked decrease in stroke volume, as well as significantly decreased cardiac output, ultimately leading to inadequate tissue perfusion.

The onset of cardiogenic shock may be abrupt or broad; however, many and varied causes have been identified. These causes can relate to interference with myocardial contractility, preload, or afterload. Causes may also be related to **hypovolemia** or various pathophysiological disorders.

Trauma-related injuries that result in cardiac tamponade, tension pneumothorax, or both can compress the myocardium and produce severe compromise in ventricular filling. Severe pulmonary embolism may contribute to poor ventricular emptying.

Cardiogenic shock is most often associated with large anterior infarctions as well as those that involve loss of more than 40 percent of the left ventricle. The mortality rate following episodes of cardiogenic shock is high, especially when dealing with geriatric patients.

Assessment of the patient in cardiogenic shock will focus on identifying the cause. Signs and symptoms will vary widely and will be based on the specific causative factor. As with all patients, it is imperative that you recognize and treat any life-threatening problems. You should also closely monitor the patient's level of consciousness, being especially attentive to alterations in mental status. In addition, an adequate patient history, if obtainable, may prove to be helpful to the patient's attending physician.

Patients in cardiogenic shock will often present with signs and symptoms of myocardial infarction. These symptoms may quickly deteriorate to manifestation of clinical evidence of severe systemic hypoperfusion. The manifestations may include:

➤ Profound hypotension (systolic BP usually less than 80 mmHg)
➤ Compensatory tachycardia
➤ Tachypnea, often resulting from associated pulmonary edema
➤ Cool, clammy skin caused by massive vasoconstriction
➤ Major dysrhythmias
➤ Respiratory difficulty
➤ Peripheral edema

Management of cardiogenic shock must be aggressive. Patients who are in cardiogenic shock should be considered seriously ill. If the patient presents in the prehospital arena, rapid transport should be quickly facilitated.

Immediate management of the patient in cardiogenic shock should be based upon the patient's clinical presentation. You should be attentive to identifying and treating the underlying cause or causes of the patient's signs and symptoms. If the patient is conscious, take care to maintain a calm demeanor and reassure the patient and his or her family.

Aggressive treatment measures may include:

➤ Airway management and ventilatory support, including administration of high-flow oxygen
➤ Circulatory support, including IV therapy
➤ Allowing the patient to assume a position of comfort, if clinically feasible
➤ EKG monitoring and treatment of presenting dysrhythmias
➤ Frequent evaluation of vital signs
➤ Pulse oximetry, to maintain O_2 saturation at 95 percent or better
➤ Medication therapy, including various vasopressors such as Dopamine, Dobutamine, and Levophed, as well as morphine sulfate, nitroglycerin, Lasix, digitalis, and sodium bicarbonate

Remember that cardiogenic shock has a relatively high mortality rate; thus the patient must be treated aggressively and immediately. You should identify and treat the underlying cause of the patient's problem and transport the patient expeditiously.

SUMMARY

Patients who experience chest pain account for the majority of all EMS calls in this country. Thousands of Americans die each year from cardiovascular emergencies, and many of these deaths occur in the prehospital arena. Cardiovascular emergencies are primarily related to obstruction of the coronary arteries due to spasm or thrombus. As health care providers, we must be able to recognize the warning signs of various cardiovascular emergencies. In addition, we must be able to intervene with appropriate and timely management.

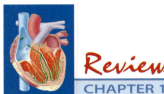

Review Questions

1. A common obstacle to the timely intervention by a health care provider when a patient complains of chest pain is:
   a. Mistrust
   b. Timidity
   c. Anxiety
   d. Denial

2. Collateral circulation allows for:
   a. Alternative path of blood flow in the event of occlusion
   b. Circulation continuum during diastole
   c. Maintaining artery patency during spasms
   d. Blood flow continuum during systole

3. The pain of angina pectoris:
   a. Is always constant
   b. Is typically temporary
   c. Occurs only during rest
   d. Is never mistaken for indigestion

4. Myocardial infarction is:
   a. Always temporary
   b. Usually diagnosed within 24 hours
   c. Age-limited in most patients
   d. Due to myocardial cell death

5. The most common cause of AMIs is:
   a. Coronary vasospasms
   b. Atherosclerotic lesions
   c. Thrombus formation
   d. Arteriosclerotic blebs

6. In acute myocardial infarctions, chest pain is:
   a. Short in duration and relieved by nitroglycerin
   b. Short in duration but not relieved by nitroglycerin
   c. Long in duration and relieved by nitroglycerin
   d. Long in duration and not relieved by nitroglycerin

7. Patients experiencing an acute myocardial infarction will always complain of chest pain.

   a. True

   b. False

8. Some elderly patients may experience an AMI without chest pain; most commonly their only presenting symptom will be a complaint of profound:

   a. Depression

   b. Weakness

   c. Nausea

   d. Dizziness

9. Unstable angina generally indicates progression of atherosclerotic heart disease and is also referred to as:

   a. PND

   b. Cor pulmonale

   c. Infarctional angina

   d. Preinfarctional angina

10. When interpreting dysrhythmias, you should remember that the most important key is the:

   a. PR interval

   b. Rate and rhythm

   c. Presence of dysrhythmias

   d. Patient's clinical appearance

11. The primary goal of management of the patient with symptomatic chest pain is to:

   a. Interrupt the infarction process

   b. Augment the infarction process

   c. Institute thrombolytic therapy

   d. Increase myocardial oxygen consumption

12. Management of a patient who is suspected of having sustained a myocardial contusion should:

   a. Focus primarily on the associated and isolated chest injury

   b. Be similar to the treatment administered to a suspected MI patient

   c. Be initiated only at the definitive care facility following transport

   d. Be completed in the prehospital arena, before transport to the hospital

13. Emergency management of left heart failure is aimed at:

   a. Decreasing myocardial oxygen demand

   b. Improving myocardial contractility

   c. Improving oxygenation and ventilation

   d. All of the above

1. Most cardiac dysrhythmias are caused by ischemia secondary to hypoxia; therefore the most appropriate drug to give a patient with any dysrhythmia is:
   a. Oxygen
   b. D5W
   c. Lidocaine
   d. Morphine

2. The fibrous sac covering the heart, which is in contact with the pleura, is the:
   a. Epicardium
   b. Myocardium
   c. Pericardium
   d. Endocardium

3. The heart ventricle with the thicker myocardium is the:
   a. Right
   b. Left

4. The pulmonic and aortic valves are open during:
   a. Systole
   b. Diastole

5. The large blood vessel that returns unoxygenated blood from the head and neck to the right atrium is called the:
   a. Jugular vein
   b. Carotid artery
   c. Superior vena cava
   d. Inferior vena cava

6. The coronary sinus, which opens into the right atrium, allows venous return from the:
   a. Azygos
   b. Pleura
   c. Myocardium
   d. Endocardium

7. The sawtooth pattern is indicative of which rhythm?
   a. Atrial fibrillation
   b. Atrial asystole
   c. Ventricular flutter
   d. None of the above

8. The mitral valve is located between the:
   a. Right and left atrium
   b. Right and left ventricle
   c. Left atrium and left ventricle
   d. Right atrium and right ventricle

9. The QRS waves of all premature complexes are usually 0.10 second or less.

    a. False

    b. True

10. The most appropriate initial w/s for defibrillating ventricular fibrillation in an adult is:

    a. 400 joules

    b. 360 joules

    c. 1 joule per kilogram

    d. 20–25 joules per kilogram

11. When preparing to defibrillate a patient who presents with ventricular fibrillation, the health care provider should do all the following except:

    a. Check pulses and lead wires

    b. Order all personnel to "stand clear"

    c. Perform cardiopulmonary resuscitation

    d. Ensure that the synchronization button is on

12. The most appropriate treatment of uncomplicated acute myocardial infarction is:

    a. IV D5W

    b. Oxygen by mask, IV LR

    c. IV NS, monitor, O_2

    d. IV D5W, monitor O_2

13. The coronary arteries receive oxygenated blood from the:

    a. Aorta

    b. Coronary sinus

    c. Pulmonary veins

    d. Pulmonary arteries

14. In the prehospital field, we administer IV fluid to a cardiac patient in order to:

    a. Provide a lifeline

    b. Allow oxygen to reach the brain

    c. Keep the patient well-hydrated

    d. Prevent incipient pump failure

15. The chambers of the heart that are thin-walled and pump against low pressure are the:

    a. Apex

    b. Aorta

    c. Atria

    d. Ventricles

16. Blood pressure is maintained by cardiac output and:

    a. Alveoli

    b. Stroke volume

    c. Coronary arteries

    d. Peripheral resistance

17. The sinoatrial node is located in the:

    a. Right atrium

    b. Right ventricle

    c. Purkinje fiber tract

    d. Atrioventricular septum

18. The AV node is located in the:

    a. Right ventricle

    b. Left ventricle

    c. Purkinje fiber tract

    d. Atrioventricular septum

19. The intrinsic firing rate of the AV node is _____ per minute.

    a. 60–100

    b. 25–35

    c. 35–45

    d. 40–60

20. The intrinsic rate of the SA node in the adult is _____ per minute.

    a. 20–60

    b. 40–80

    c. 60–100

    d. 80–100

21. The electrocardiogram is used to:

    a. Determine pulse rate

    b. Detect valvular dysfunction

    c. Evaluate electrical activity in the heart

    d. Determine whether the heart muscle is contracting

22. The PR interval should normally be _____ second or smaller.

    a. 0.10

    b. 0.12

    c. 0.08

    d. 0.20

23. The QRS interval should normally be _____ second or smaller.

    a. 0.20

    b. 0.12

    c. 0.18

    d. 0.36

24. The heart has four chambers; the upper chambers are called:

    a. Atria

    b. Ventricles

    c. Septa

    d. Branches

25. A sinus rhythm with cyclic variation caused by alterations in the respiratory pattern is:

    a. Sinus arrest

    b. Sinus tachycardia

    c. Sinus dysrhythmia

    d. Supraventricular dysrhythmia

26. A sudden (paroxysmal) onset of tachycardia with a stimulus that arises above the AV node refers to a:

    a. Sinus arrest

    b. Sinus tachycardia

    c. Sinus dysrhythmia

    d. Supraventricular dysrhythmia

27. Oscilloscopic evidence of ventricular fibrillation can be mimicked by artifact.

    a. True

    b. False

28. In the presence of ventricular fibrillation, attempts at countershock might be ineffective because of:

    a. Metabolic acidosis

    b. Ventricular irritability

    c. Inadequate oxygenation

    d. All of the above

29. Before performing carotid sinus massage, you should do all the following except:

    a. Monitor the EKG

    b. Ensure that the carotid pulses are present

    c. Have the patient perform Valsalva's maneuver

    d. Establish a secure airway by intubating the trachea

30. The QRS complex is produced when the:
    a. Ventricles repolarize
    b. Ventricles depolarize
    c. Ventricles contract
    d. Both b and c

31. Most atrial fibrillation waves are not followed by a QRS complex because the:
    a. Impulses are initiated in the left ventricle
    b. Stimuli are not strong enough to be conducted
    c. Ventricle can receive only 120 stimuli in 1 minute
    d. AV junction is unable to conduct all the excitation impulses

32. Identify the normal impulse flow of the heart's electrical conduction system:
    1. SA node
    2. Purkinje fibers
    3. Bundle of His
    4. AV node
    5. Bundle branches
    6. Internodal pathways
    a. 1, 5, 2, 4, 6, 3
    b. 1, 6, 4, 3, 5, 2
    c. 1, 4, 3, 6, 5, 2
    d. 1, 2, 3, 4, 5, 6

33. When the EKG shows no relationship between the P wave and the QRS complex, you should suspect:
    a. First-degree block
    b. Second-degree block
    c. Third-degree block
    d. Electromechanical dissociation

34. The pain of stable angina pectoris is:
    a. Predictable
    b. Not predictable
    c. Never very severe
    d. Usually undetectable

35. Signs and symptoms that may be observed in a patient with necrotic heart tissue could include:
    a. Dysrhythmias
    b. Congestive heart failure
    c. Cardiogenic shock (severe)
    d. All of the above

36. The term "supraventricular" indicates a stimulus arising above the ventricles.
    a. True
    b. False

37. Wenckebach differs from complete heart block in that CHB has a:
    a. Faster rate
    b. Normal QRS
    c. Constant PR interval
    d. Regular R-R interval

38. PAT is a sudden onset of atrial tachycardia.
    a. True
    b. False

39. The T wave on the EKG strip represents:
    a. Rest period
    b. Bundle of His
    c. Atrial contraction
    d. Ventricular contraction

40. The coronary circulation has how many main arteries?
    a. Two
    b. Six
    c. Four
    d. Eight

41. Starling's law may be expressed as follows:
    a. An increase in systolic filling does not alter cardiac output.
    b. A decrease in systolic filling will decrease the force of contraction.
    c. An increase in diastolic filling will increase the force of contraction.
    d. An increase in filling time yields greater cardiac output regardless of peripheral resistance.

42. PEA or pulseless electrical activity may be manifested by a:
    a. Normal EKG, normal pulse
    b. Normal EKG, absent pulse
    c. Abnormal EKG, normal pulse
    d. Abnormal EKG, absent pulse

43. The function of the chordae tendineae and papillary muscles is to:
    a. Prevent backflow of blood into the ventricles
    b. Protect the coronary orifices when the aortic valve opens
    c. Prevent backflow of blood into the atrium
    d. Facilitate backflow of blood from the aorta

44. A 50-year-old man is complaining of chest pain that began while he was clearing underbrush on a vacant lot. He describes the pain as a "heavy pressure" which has lasted 5–10 minutes. V/S are: 140/95, HR: 82, R: 16. He has no previous cardiac history. EKG shows NSR. The chest pain is most probably due to:
    a. Dysrhythmias
    b. Pulmonary embolus
    c. Coronary insufficiency
    d. Congestive heart failure

45. Lead II is most commonly used in the prehospital arena because it:
    a. Is easier to apply
    b. Shows good T waves
    c. Illustrates good P waves
    d. Is faster to apply

46. The ability of certain cardiac cells to initiate excitation impulses spontaneously is called:
    a. Automaticity
    b. Contractility
    c. Conductivity
    d. Excitability

47. The keys to interpretation of second-degree heart block, Mobitz type II, are the presence of constant PR intervals and the fact that there are more P waves present than QRS complexes.
    a. True
    b. False

48. The absence of electrical impulse results in the recording of a flat line on an EKG strip.
    a. False
    b. True

49. Your patient is a driver who was in a head-on automobile collision. Upon arrival at the patient's side you immediately notice that the steering wheel is bent and that the patient has multiple contusions on the chest area. You realize you are probably dealing with:
    a. Angina pectoris
    b. A drunk patient
    c. Myocardial trauma
    d. Hypertensive crisis

50. A man complains of substernal chest pain radiating to his left arm and jaw. He has vomited once and still feels nauseated. He is sitting up, appears to be short of breath, and is sweating profusely. Your patient's symptoms most probably are related to:
    a. Pacemaker failure
    b. Pulmonary edema
    c. Hypertensive crisis
    d. Acute myocardial infarction

51. If a known coronary bypass patient suffers a cardiac arrest, the health care provider should:
    a. Not perform CPR, because of the risk of further injury
    b. Deliver lighter compressions, because of the risk of further injury
    c. Provide CPR in the same manner as for any other patient in arrest
    d. Provide CPR unless fracture of the sternum or ribs becomes apparent

52. The expected rate of a junctional escape rhythm is _____ bpm.
    a. 20–40
    b. 60–100
    c. 40–60
    d. 60–80

53. When interpreting dysrhythmias, you should remember that the most important key is the:
    a. PR interval
    b. Rate and rhythm
    c. Presence of dysrhythmias
    d. Patient's clinical appearance

54. In order to obtain a two-lead EKG strip, you should apply _____ leads to the patient's chest.
    a. Three
    b. Four
    c. Five
    d. Six

55. The uppermost portion of the heart is known as the:
    a. Apex
    b. Base
    c. Atria
    d. Aorta

56. The most common causes of poor EKG tracings are:
    a. Patient movement
    b. Loose leads/electrodes
    c. Both a and b
    d. None of the above

57. "A graphic record of the electrical activity of the heart" describes a(an):
    a. Echocardiogram
    b. Electrocardiogram
    c. Encephalogram
    d. Radiogram

58. The primary treatment for multifocal PVCs is:
    a. Defibrillation
    b. Cardioversion
    c. Oxygen administration
    d. None of the above

59. In order to calculate heart rate accurately by the R-to-R interval method, the patient must have a regular rhythm.
    a. True
    b. False

60. Second-degree heart block, type I, may be transient and self-correcting.
    a. True
    b. False

61. Cardiovascular disease is the number one cause of death in the United States.
    a. False
    b. True

62. Prompt, definitive intervention has proved effective in preventing many deaths from cardiovascular disease.
    a. True
    b. False

63. The innermost lining of the heart is contiguous with the visceral pericardium and is called the:
    a. Endocardium
    b. Pericardium
    c. Myocardium
    d. Epicardium

64. The right and left atria are separated anatomically by the:
    a. Interatrial septum
    b. Bundle of Kent
    c. Interventricular septum
    d. Endocardial mass

65. The right atrium receives blood from the myocardium via the:
    a. Left marginal branch
    b. Inferior vena cava
    c. Great cardiac vein
    d. Internal carotid artery

66. Two examples of atrioventricular valves are:
    1. Pulmonic valve
    2. Tricuspid valve
    3. Papillary valve
    4. Bicuspid valve
    a. 1 and 2
    b. 2 and 4
    c. 1 and 3
    d. 3 and 4

67. Deoxygenated blood enters the heart through the:
    1. Coronary sinus
    2. Pulmonary artery
    3. Superior vena cava
    4. Inferior vena cava
    a. 1, 2, and 3
    b. 2, 3, and 4
    c. 2 and 3 only
    d. 1, 3, and 4

68. In EKG strips representing dysrhythmias originating in the AV junction, the P wave, if present, will be inverted or absent.
    a. True
    b. False

69. The amount of blood ejected by the heart in one cardiac contraction is known as:
    a. Preload
    b. Afterload
    c. Cardiac cycle
    d. Stroke volume

70. The pressure in the ventricle at the end of diastole is referred to as:

    a. Preload

    b. Afterload

    c. Cardiac output

    d. Autonomic

71. The parasympathetic nervous system is mediated by the tenth cranial nerve, which runs from the brain stem to the rectum. This nerve is called the:

    a. Optic

    b. Vagus

    c. Plexus

    d. Ganglia

72. The neurotransmitter for the parasympathetic nervous system is acetylcholine. Release of acetylcholine:

    1. Slows the heart rate

    2. Increases the heart rate

    3. Slows atrioventricular conduction

    4. Increases atrioventricular conduction

    a. 1 and 3

    b. 2 and 3

    c. 3 and 4

    d. 1 and 4

73. Hyperkalemia refers to an increased level of potassium in the blood and can result in decreased automaticity and conduction.

    a. True

    b. False

74. Cardiac function, both electrical and mechanical, is strongly influenced by electrolyte imbalance.

    a. True

    b. False

75. An EKG strip illustrates a regular rhythm, a heart rate of 70, and QRS complexes that are within normal limits. P waves are variable in configuration across the strip. This rhythm is identified as a:

    a. Wandering atrial pacemaker

    b. First-degree heart block

    c. Third-degree heart block

    d. Second-degree heart block, Mobitz I

76.   Ventricular irritability in the presence of myocardial infarction is:

    a.   A precursor to respiratory involvement

    b.   Very dangerous and should be treated

    c.   To be expected and not a cause for alarm

    d.   Highly unlikely if oxygen is administered

77.   Prolonged episodes of SVT may increase myocardial oxygen demand and may thus increase the need for supplemental oxygen therapy.

    a.   True

    b.   False

78.   A progressing PR interval until such time as that a QRS is dropped is considered to be:

    a.   Third-degree block

    b.   Atrial fibrillation

    c.   Second-degree AV block, Mobitz type I

    d.   Second-degree AV block, Mobitz type II

79.   Artifact is defined as EKG waveforms produced from sources outside the heart.

    a.   True

    b.   False

80.   Parasympathetic stimulation controls cardiac action by reducing the heart rate, the speed of impulse through the AV node, and the force of atrial contraction. This response is known as the:

    a.   Nodal response

    b.   SA node

    c.   Neurotransmitter

    d.   Vagal response

81.   An abnormality in conduction through the ventricles may be identified on the EKG tracing by a(an):

    a.   Distorted, varying P-wave pattern

    b.   Prolonged PR interval

    c.   Wide and bizarre QRS complex

    d.   Elevated S-T segment

82.   All the following statements regarding premature ventricular complexes (PVCs) are true except:

    a.   Occasional PVCs may occur in persons without heart disease.

    b.   Bursts of two or more PVCs in a row may progress rapidly to ventricular tachycardia.

    c.   A PVC falling on a T wave may cause ventricular fibrillation.

    d.   Frequent PVCs in a patient without heart disease require no treatment.

83. Lidocaine should be considered for suppressing premature ventricular contractions (PVCs) in acute myocardial infarction in which situation?

    a. When the PVCs are more frequent than six per minute or are multifocal

    b. In second- or third-degree heart block

    c. In the presence of sinus bradycardia

    d. With a patient who is known to be allergic to local anesthetics

84. The term for the condition in which there are regular ventricular complexes on the EKG monitor but no palpable pulse is:

    a. Pacemaker rhythm

    b. Vagal response

    c. Mechanical CPR

    d. Pulseless electrical activity

85. The pause following an ectopic beat where the SA node is unaffected and the cadence of the heart is uninterrupted is called:

    a. Asynchronous

    b. Noncompensatory

    c. Interpolated

    d. Compensatory

86. The faster discharging rate of the AV junction in an accelerated junctional rhythm may be due to:

    a. Increased automaticity of the AV junction

    b. Blockage of the parasympathetic nervous system response

    c. Increased excitation of the internodal pathways

    d. Increased excitation of the sinoatrial node

87. Paroxysmal junctional tachycardia is often more appropriately called paroxysmal supraventricular tachycardia, since it may be difficult to distinguish this rhythm from paroxysmal atrial tachycardia due to the rapid rate.

    a. True

    b. False

88. Vagal maneuvers are commonly used to treat:

    a. Ventricular tachycardia

    b. Paroxysmal junctional tachycardia

    c. Paroxysmal supraventricular tachycardia

    d. B and c only

89. All the following are true of third-degree AV block except:

    a. The atria and the ventricles pace the heart independent of each other.

    b. Both the atrial and the ventricular rates are usually regular.

    c. There is no relationship between P waves and R waves.

    d. Although the atria and ventricles are disassociated, their rates are generally the same.

90. Defibrillation is the treatment of choice for:

    1. Asystole
    2. Pulseless ventricular tachycardia
    3. Ventricular fibrillation
    4. Idioventricular rhythms

    a. 1, 2, and 3
    b. 2 and 3
    c. 1, 3, and 4
    d. 3 and 4

91. A ventricular escape beat or ventricular escape rhythm results when:

    1. The vagus nerve is hyperstimulated
    2. Impulses from higher pacemakers fail to reach the ventricles
    3. A ventricular excitation impulse escapes from the AV junction
    4. The rate of discharge of higher pacemakers becomes less than that of the ventricles.

    a. 1 and 3
    b. 2 and 4
    c. 1, 2, and 3
    d. 2, 3, and 4

92. Since unifocal PVCs imply uniform irritability of the entire myocardium, they are generally considered more life-threatening than multifocal PVCs.

    a. True
    b. False

93. A 69-year-old man is experiencing mild chest pain. Physical exam reveals no other significant findings. Vital signs are: BP = 160/88, pulse = 84 and irregular, respirations = 24. Cardiac monitor reveals a normal sinus rhythm with five unifocal PVCs per minute. The most appropriate prehospital treatment is:

    a. Monitor patient only—no treatment necessary
    b. Oxygen at 4 liters per nasal cannula; IV with D5W at KVO rate; cardiac monitor
    c. Oxygen at 10 liters per endotracheal tube; rapid IV infusion of RL; cardiac monitor
    d. Oxygen via nonrebreathing mask; IV; cardiac monitor; immediate transport to hospital

94. Which of the following is *not* a trait of malignant or dangerous PVCs?

    a. Unifocal premature complexes
    b. R on T phenomenon
    c. Greater than six per minute
    d. Runs of ventricular tachycardia

95. All the following are treatments for ventricular fibrillation:

    1. Intubate
    2. Begin CPR
    3. Defibrillate at 360 joules
    4. Establish IV access

    The correct sequence for these treatments is:

    a. 2, 3, 1, 4
    b. 1, 2, 3, 4
    c. 4, 3, 1, 2
    d. 3, 2, 1, 4

96. Your patient is an 82-year-old woman with a history of coronary artery disease. She is conscious and alert. She is complaining of substernal chest pain, radiating into the left arm. She is diaphoretic and short of breath. BP = 120/64, pulse is 56 and irregular, respirations are 32, shallow and congested. You connect the cardiac monitor, and it shows ventricular fibrillation. Your immediate action is to:

    a. Begin CPR
    b. Prepare to defibrillate at 200 joules
    c. Check the monitor leads
    d. Defibrillate at 360 joules

97. You observe an EKG pattern of "irregular irregularity" on an EKG strip. This strip probably represents:

    a. Atrial flutter
    b. Atrial fibrillation
    c. Atrial tachycardia
    d. Ventricular pacemaker

98. Since pacemakers are susceptible to damage from strong electrical stimuli, you should never defibrillate a patient who has an implanted pacemaker at a setting over 300 joules.

    a. True
    b. False

99. A first-degree AV block is a delay in conduction at the level of the AV node rather than an actual block.

    a. True
    b. False

100. Second-degree AV block (Mobitz II) is usually associated with acute myocardial infarction and septal necrosis and is considered to be more serious than Wenckebach.

    a. True
    b. False

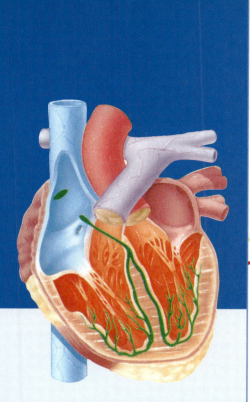

chapter 15

Review EKG Strips

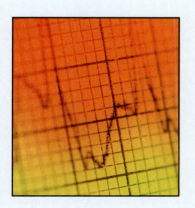

INTRODUCTION

This chapter is included in order to provide review strips that will reinforce your newly acquired knowledge of EKG interpretation. I encourage you to apply the five-step approach to interpret each of the following rhythm strips.

When you have completed this chapter, check your answers with the answers provided in Appendix 2. It should not be assumed that all strips are 6-second strips. You should carefully count the seconds in each strip, so that you will reinforce your interpretative skills.

Good luck! Enjoy applying your newly acquired EKG interpretive skills to interpret these review strips.

Note:

➤ "Rate" and "rhythm" refer to ventricular rate and rhythm, unless otherwise noted.

➤ A denotes "absent".

➤ I denotes " indistinguishable".

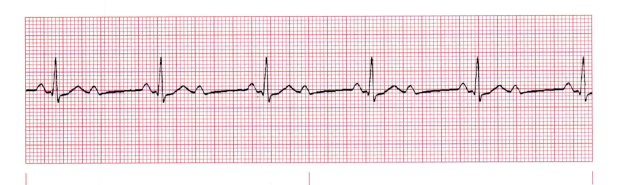

1. Rate: _____   Rhythm: _____
   P wave: _____   PRI: _____
   QRS complex: _____   Interpretation: _____

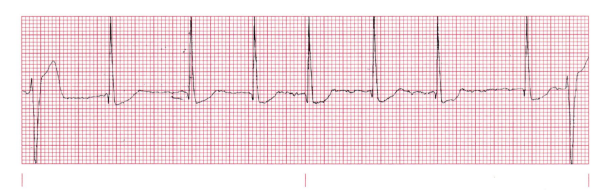

2. Rate: _____   Rhythm: _____
   P wave: _____   PRI: _____
   QRS complex: _____   Interpretation: _____

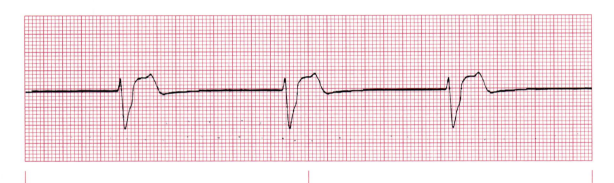

3. Rate: _____   Rhythm: _____
   P wave: _____   PRI: _____
   QRS complex: _____   Interpretation: _____

4. Rate: _____   Rhythm:_____
P wave: _____   PRI: _____
QRS complex: _____   Interpretation: _____

5. Rate: _____   Rhythm:_____
P wave: _____   PRI: _____
QRS complex: _____   Interpretation: _____

6. Rate: _____   Rhythm:_____
P wave: _____   PRI: _____
QRS complex: _____   Interpretation: _____

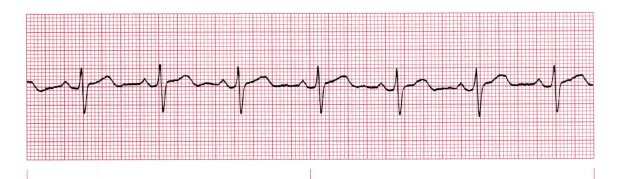

7. Rate: _____   Rhythm: _____

    P wave: _____   PRI: _____

    QRS complex: _____   Interpretation: _____

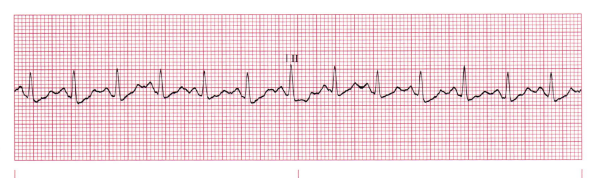

8. Rate: _____   Rhythm: _____

    P wave: _____   PRI: _____

    QRS complex: _____   Interpretation: _____

9. Rate: _____   Rhythm: _____

    P wave: _____   PRI: _____

    QRS complex: _____   Interpretation: _____

10. Rate: _____   Rhythm:_____

P wave: _____   PRI: _____

QRS complex: _____   Interpretation: _____

11. Rate: _____   Rhythm:_____

P wave: _____   PRI: _____

QRS complex: _____   Interpretation: _____

12. Rate: _____   Rhythm:_____

P wave: _____   PRI: _____

QRS complex: _____   Interpretation: _____

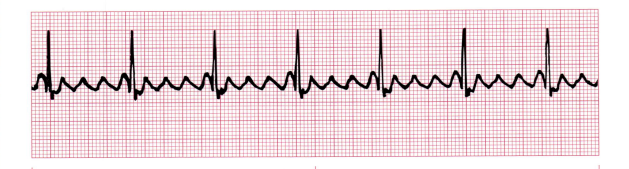

13. Rate: _____ Rhythm: _____
   P wave: _____ PRI: _____
   QRS complex: _____ Interpretation: _____

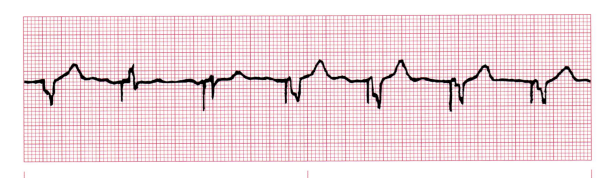

14. Rate: _____ Rhythm: _____
   P wave: _____ PRI: _____
   QRS complex: _____ Interpretation: _____

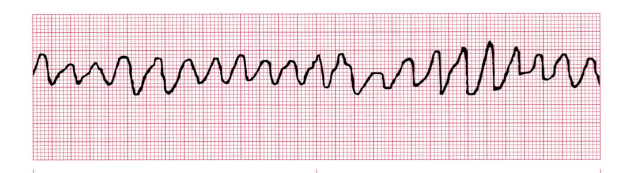

15. Rate: _____ Rhythm: _____
   P wave: _____ PRI: _____
   QRS complex: _____ Interpretation: _____

16. Rate: _____   Rhythm:_____
    P wave: _____   PRI: _____
    QRS complex: _____   Interpretation: _____

17. Rate: _____   Rhythm:_____
    P wave: _____   PRI: _____
    QRS complex: _____   Interpretation: _____

18. Rate: _____   Rhythm:_____
    P wave: _____   PRI: _____
    QRS complex: _____   Interpretation: _____

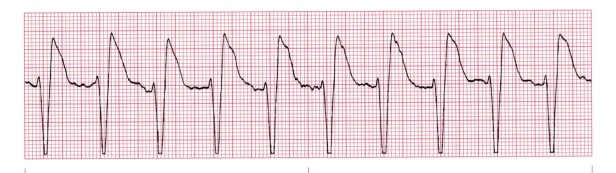

19. Rate: _____   Rhythm:_____
    P wave: _____   PRI: _____
    QRS complex: _____   Interpretation: _____

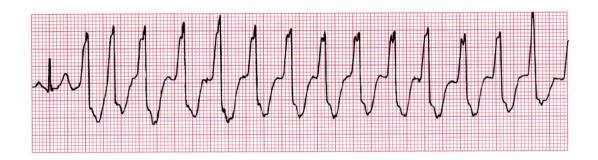

20. Rate: _____   Rhythm:_____
    P wave: _____   PRI: _____
    QRS complex: _____   Interpretation: _____

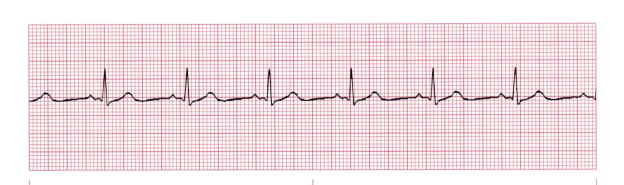

21. Rate: _____   Rhythm:_____
    P wave: _____   PRI: _____
    QRS complex: _____   Interpretation: _____

22. Rate: _____   Rhythm:_____

P wave: _____   PRI: _____

QRS complex: _____   Interpretation: _____

23. Rate: _____   Rhythm:_____

P wave: _____   PRI: _____

QRS complex: _____   Interpretation: _____

24. Rate: _____   Rhythm:_____

P wave: _____   PRI: _____

QRS complex: _____   Interpretation: _____

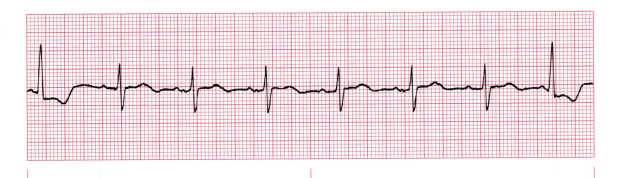

25. Rate: _____ Rhythm: _____

P wave: _____ PRI: _____

QRS complex: _____ Interpretation: _____

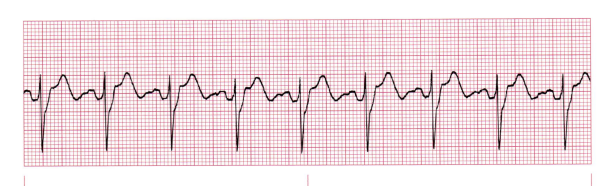

26. Rate: _____ Rhythm: _____

P wave: _____ PRI: _____

QRS complex: _____ Interpretation: _____

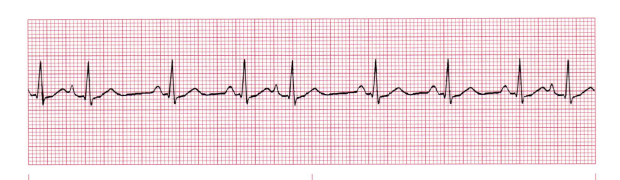

27. Rate: _____ Rhythm: _____

P wave: _____ PRI: _____

QRS complex: _____ Interpretation: _____

28. Rate: _____   Rhythm:_____

    P wave: _____   PRI: _____

    QRS complex: _____   Interpretation: _____

29. Rate: _____   Rhythm:_____

    P wave: _____   PRI: _____

    QRS complex: _____   Interpretation: _____

30. Rate: _____   Rhythm:_____

    P wave: _____   PRI: _____

    QRS complex: _____   Interpretation: _____

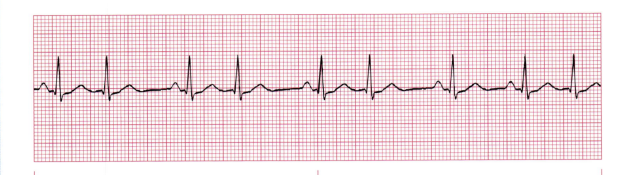

31. Rate: _____   Rhythm:_____

P wave: _____   PRI: _____

QRS complex: _____   Interpretation: _____

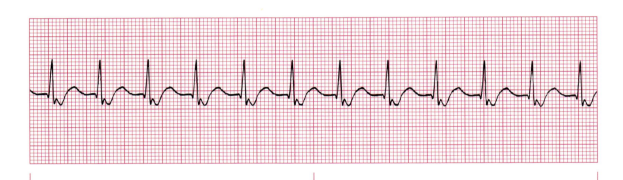

32. Rate: _____   Rhythm:_____

P wave: _____   PRI: _____

QRS complex: _____   Interpretation: _____

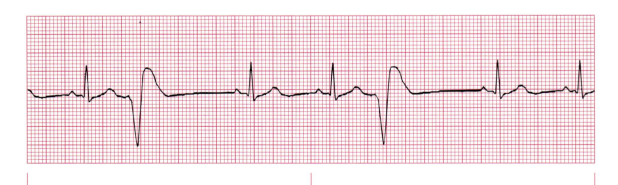

33. Rate: _____   Rhythm:_____

P wave: _____   PRI: _____

QRS complex: _____   Interpretation: _____

34. Rate: _____   Rhythm:_____

P wave: _____   PRI: _____

QRS complex: _____   Interpretation: _____

35. Rate: _____   Rhythm:_____

P wave: _____   PRI: _____

QRS complex: _____   Interpretation: _____

36. Rate: _____   Rhythm:_____

P wave: _____   PRI: _____

QRS complex: _____   Interpretation: _____

37. Rate: _____   Rhythm: _____

P wave: _____   PRI: _____

QRS complex: _____   Interpretation: _____

38. Rate: _____   Rhythm: _____

P wave: _____   PRI: _____

QRS complex: _____   Interpretation: _____

39. Rate: _____   Rhythm: _____

P wave: _____   PRI: _____

QRS complex: _____   Interpretation: _____

40. Rate: _____   Rhythm: _____

P wave: _____   PRI: _____

QRS complex: _____   Interpretation: _____

41. Rate: _____   Rhythm: _____

P wave: _____   PRI: _____

QRS complex: _____   Interpretation: _____

42. Rate: _____   Rhythm: _____

P wave: _____   PRI: _____

QRS complex: _____   Interpretation: _____

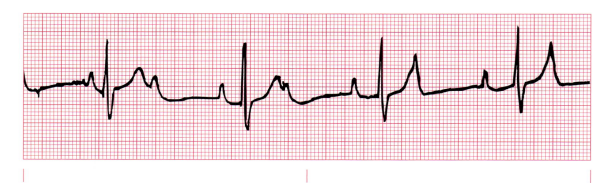

49. Rate: _____ Rhythm:_____

P wave: _____ PRI: _____

QRS complex: _____ Interpretation: _____

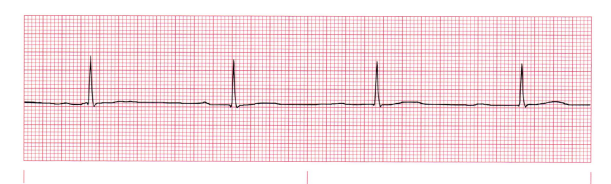

50. Rate: _____ Rhythm:_____

P wave: _____ PRI: _____

QRS complex: _____ Interpretation: _____

Appendix 1

ANSWERS TO REVIEW QUESTIONS

CHAPTERS 1–14

CHAPTER 1

1. c
2. b
3. a
4. c
5. a
6. b
7. d
8. c
9. b
10. c
11. b
12. a
13. d
14. b
15. c

CHAPTER 2

1. a
2. b
3. b
4. d
5. a
6. c
7. b
8. d
9. a
10. b
11. c
12. d
13. c
14. d
15. a

CHAPTER 3

1. c
2. a
3. a
4. d
5. a
6. d
7. a
8. a

9. a
10. a
11. c
12. a
13. b
14. c
15. d

CHAPTER 4

1. a
2. a
3. d
4. c
5. c
6. b
7. c
8. c

9. b
10. c
11. b
12. a
13. b
14. c
15. c

CHAPTER 5

1. b
2. c
3. d
4. b
5. d
6. b
7. a
8. a

9. d
10. b
11. a
12. a
13. c
14. a
15. a

CHAPTER 6

1. b
2. d
3. a
4. c
5. d
6. b
7. a
8. d

9. b
10. a
11. a
12. d
13. a
14. b
15. a

CHAPTER 7 (REVIEW QUESTIONS)

1. c
2. b
3. a
4. d
5. d
6. a
7. b
8. a

9. b
10. d
11. a
12. a
13. a
14. a
15. a

CHAPTER 7 (REVIEW STRIPS)

1. Rate: 75
    P wave: Present and upright
    QRS: 0.06
    Rhythm: Regular
    PRI: 0.24
    Interpretation: Normal sinus rhythm

2. Rate: 107
    P wave: Present and upright
    QRS: 0.08
    Rhythm: Regular
    PRI: 0.16
    Interpretation: Sinus tachycardia

3. Rate: 50
    P wave: Present and upright
    QRS: 0.08
    Rhythm: Regular
    PRI: 0.14
    Interpretation: Sinus bradycardia

4. Rate: 70
    P wave: Present and upright
    QRS: 0.08
    Rhythm: Irregular
    PRI: 0.16
    Interpretation: Sinus dysrhythmia

5. Rate: 40
    P wave: Present and upright
    QRS: 0.06
    Rhythm: Irregular
    PRI: 0.16
    Interpretation: Sinus brady with sinus arrest

6. Rate: 70
    P wave: Present and upright
    QRS: 0.08
    Rhythm: Irregular
    PRI: 0.16
    Interpretation: Sinus dysrhythmia

7. Rate: 136
    P wave: Present and upright
    QRS: 0.06
    Rhythm: Regular
    PRI: 0.18
    Interpretation: Sinus tachycardia

8. Rate: 80
    P wave: Present and upright
    QRS: 0.04
    Rhythm: Irregular
    PRI: 0.16
    Interpretation: Sinus dysrhythmia

9. Rate: 50
    P wave: Present and upright
    QRS: 0.08
    Rhythm: Regular
    PRI: 0.14
    Interpretation: Sinus bradycardia

10. Rate: 60
    P wave: Present and upright
    QRS: 0.08
    Rhythm: Irregular
    PRI: 0.16
    Interpretation: Sinus arrest rhythm

CHAPTER 8

1. a
2. a
3. b
4. d
5. c
6. d
7. a
8. a
9. a
10. d
11. a
12. b
13. c
14. b,
15. d

CHAPTER 8 (REVIEW STRIPS)

1. Rate: 50
   P wave: Present and upright with varying morphology
   QRS: 0.04
   Rhythm: Regular
   PRI: varies
   Interpretation: Wandering atrial pacemaker

2. Rate: 80
   P wave: Flutter waves
   QRS: 0.06
   Rhythm: Regular
   PRI: Indistinguishable (I)
   Interpretation: Atrial flutter: 4:1 ratio

3. Rate: 60
   P wave: f waves
   QRS: 0.08
   Rhythm: Irregularly irregular
   PRI: Indistinguishable
   Interpretation: Atrial fibrillation

4. Rate: 70
   P wave: Present and upright
   QRS: 0.06
   Rhythm: Irregular
   PRI: 0.16
   Interpretation: Sinus rhythm with PACs

5. Rate: 210
   P wave: Indistinguishable
   QRS: 0.06
   Rhythm: Regular
   PRI: I
   Interpretation: Supraventricular tachycardia

6. Rate: 50
   P wave: I
   QRS: 0.06
   Rhythm: Irregularly irregular
   PRI: I
   Interpretation: Atrial fibrillation

7. Rate: 80
   P wave: Present and upright
   QRS: 0.10
   Rhythm: Irregular
   PRI: 0.14
   Interpretation: Sinus rhythm with a PAC

8. Rate: 90
   P wave: Flutter waves
   QRS: 0.06
   Rhythm: Irregular
   PRI: I
   Interpretation: Atrial flutter: variable ventricular response

9. Rate: 190
   P wave: I
   QRS: 0.08
   Rhythm: Regular
   PRI: I
   Interpretation: Supraventricular tachycardia

10. Rate: 50
    P wave: Varying morphology
    QRS: 0.06
    Rhythm: Regular
    PRI: Variable
    Interpretation: Wandering atrial pacemaker

CHAPTER 9

1. a	9. b
2. d	10. d
3. c	11. a
4. d	12. d
5. c	13. a
6. a	14. a
7. c	15. a
8. c	

CHAPTER 9 (REVIEW STRIPS)

1. Rate: 70 — Rhythm: Regular
    P wave: Present and inverted — PRI: 0.10
    QRS: 0.06 — Interpretation: Accelerated junctional rhythm

2. Rate: 30 — Rhythm: Regular
    P wave: A — PRI: A
    QRS: 0.06 — Interpretation: Junctional rhythm

3. Rate: 70 — Rhythm: Irregular
    P wave: Present and upright — PRI: 0.14
    except for ectopic beat
    QRS: 0.10 — Interpretation: Sinus rhythm with PJCs

4. Rate: 120 — Rhythm: Regular
    P wave: A — PRI: A
    QRS: 0.08 — Interpretation: Junctional tachycardia

5. Rate: 70 — Rhythm: Irregular
    P wave: Present and upright — PRI: 0.16
    except for ectopic beats
    QRS: 0.08 — Interpretation: Sinus rhythm with PJCs
    (bigeminy)

6. Rate: 70 — Rhythm: Regular
    P wave: A — PRI: A
    QRS: 0.06 — Interpretation: Accelerated junctional rhythm

7. Rate: 40 — Rhythm: Regular
    P wave: Inverted, follow QRS — PRI: A
    QRS: 0.08 — Interpretation: Junctional rhythm

8. Rate: 120 — Rhythm: Regular
    P wave: A — PRI: A
    QRS: 0.10 — Interpretation: Junctional tachycardia

CHAPTER 10

1. c
2. a
3. d
4. c
5. b
6. b
7. a
8. b

9. a
10. a
11. a
12. c
13. a
14. c
15. d

CHAPTER 10 (REVIEW STRIPS)

1. Rate: I
   P wave: A
   QRS: A

   Rhythm: I
   PRI: A
   Interpretation: Coarse ventricular fibrillation

2. Rate: I
   P wave: A
   QRS: A

   Rhythm: I
   PRI: A
   Interpretation: Fine ventricular fibrillation

3. Rate: A
   P wave: A
   QRS: A

   Rhythm: A
   PRI: A
   Interpretation: Asystole

4. Rate: Atrial rate: 40
   P wave: Present and upright
   QRS: A

   Rhythm: Atrial rhythm: regular
   PRI: A
   Interpretation: Ventricular asystole

5. Rate: 140
   P wave: A
   QRS: 0.28

   Rhythm: Regular
   PRI: A
   Interpretation: Ventricular tachycardia

6. Rate: 110
   P wave: Present and upright
   QRS: 0.06

   Rhythm: Irregular
   PRI: 0.16
   Interpretation: Sinus rhythm with quadrigeminy

7. Rate: 120
   P wave: Present upright except for ectopic beats
   QRS: 0.06

   Rhythm: Irregular
   PRI: 0.16

   Interpretation: Sinus rhythm with couplet PVCs

8. Rate: 80
   P wave: Present and upright except for ectopic beats
   QRS: 0.04

   Rhythm: Irregular
   PRI: 0.12

   Interpretation: Sinus rhythm with multifocal PVCs

9. Rate: 70
   P wave: Present and upright except for ectopic beats
   QRS: 0.08

   Rhythm: Irregular
   PRI: 0.20

   Interpretation: Sinus rhythm with unifocal PVCs

10. Rate: I   Rhythm: I
    P wave: A   PRI: A
    QRS: A   Interpretation: Torsades de pointes

11. Rate: 190   Rhythm: Regular
    P wave: A   PRI: A
    QRS: 0.16   Interpretation: Ventricular tachycardia

12. Rate: 70   Rhythm: Irregular
    P wave: Present and upright   PRI: 0.18
    except for ectopic beats
    QRS: 0.08   Interpretation: Sinus rhythm with unifocal
                                     PVCs

13. Rate: 80   Rhythm: Irregular
    P wave: Present and upright   PRI: 0.16
    except for ectopic beats
    QRS: 0.08   Interpretation: Sinus rhythm with unifocal
                                     PVCs (bigeminy)

14. Rate: 40   Rhythm: Regular
    P wave: A   PRI: A
    QRS: 0.16   Interpretation: Idioventricular rhythm

CHAPTER 11

1. c	9. c
2. d	10. c
3. a	11. a
4. a	12. a
5. a	13. a
6. d	14. a
7. a	15. a
8. b	

CHAPTER 11 (REVIEW STRIPS)

1. Rate: 60   Rhythm: Regular
   P wave: Present and upright   PRI: Varies
   QRS: 0.08   Interpretation: Third-degree heart block

2. Rate: 70   Rhythm: Regular
   P wave: Present and upright   PRI: 0.22
   QRS: 0.06   Interpretation: First-degree heart block

3. Rate: 60   Rhythm: Regular
   P wave: Present and upright   PRI: Varies
   QRS: 0.08   Interpretation: Third-degree heart block

4. Rate: 70
   P wave: Present and upright

   QRS: 0.08

   Rhythm: Irregular
   PRI: Progressively prolonging until QRS is dropped
   Interpretation: Second-degree heart block, Mobitz type I; Wenchebach

5. Rate: 60
   P wave: Present and upright
   QRS: 0.08

   Rhythm: Regular
   PRI: 0.28
   Interpretation: First-degree heart block

6. Rate: 20
   P wave: Present and upright
   QRS: 0.12

   Rhythm: Regular
   PRI: Variable
   Interpretation: Third-degree heart block

7. Rate: 40
   P wave: Present and upright
   QRS: 0.12

   Rhythm: Regular
   PRI: 0.24
   Interpretation: Second-degree block, type II, 2:1 conduction

8. Rate: 60
   P wave: Present and upright

   QRS: 0.08

   Rhythm: Irregular
   PRI: Progressively prolonging, until QRS is dropped
   Interpretation: Second-degree heart block, Mobitz type I; Wenchebach

CHAPTER 12

1. a
2. b
3. a
4. c
5. b
6. a
7. a
8. a

9. b
10. d
11. a
12. a
13. a
14. a
15. a

CHAPTER 12 (REVIEW STRIPS)

1. Rate: 40
   P wave: Varies
   QRS: 0.12

   Rhythm: Regular
   PRI: Varies
   Interpretation: Malfunctioning pacemaker and third-degree block

2. Rate: 80
   P wave: Generated by pacer
   QRS: 0.16

   Rhythm: Regular
   PRI: 0.14
   Interpretation: Sequential AV pacemaker rhythm

3. Rate: 80
   P wave: Present and upright in normal complexes
   QRS: 0.04

   Rhythm: Irregular
   PRI: 0.16

   Interpretation: Sinus rhythm with ventricular demand pacer

4. Rate: 70   Rhythm: Regular
   P wave: A   PRI: A
   QRS: 0.14   Interpretation: Ventricular pacemaker rhythm

5. Rate: 90   Rhythm: Regular
   P wave: A   PRI: A
   QRS: 0.14   Interpretation: Ventricular pacemaker rhythm

6. Rate: 50   Rhythm: Irregular
   P wave: Present and upright   PRI: 0.24
   QRS: 0.08   Interpretation: Malfunctioning pacemaker
                                     rhythm; first-degree heart block

7. Rate: 70   Rhythm: Regular
   P wave: A   PRI: A
   QRS: 0.12   Interpretation: Ventricular pacemaker rhythm

8. Rate: 80   Rhythm: Irregular
   P wave: A   PRI: A
   QRS: 0.12   Interpretation: Malfunctioning pacemaker
                       rhythm

CHAPTER 13

1. d	11. a
2. a	12. b
3. b	13. d
4. d	14. d
5. c	15. c
6. d	16. c
7. b	17. b
8. b	18. a
9. d	19. c
10. d	20. a

CHAPTER 14

1. a	15. c
2. c	16. d
3. b	17. a
4. a	18. d
5. c	19. d
6. c	20. c
7. d	21. c
8. c	22. d
9. a	23. b
10. b	24. a
11. d	25. c
12. c	26. d
13. a	27. a
14. a	28. d

29.	d	65.	c
30.	d	66.	b
31.	d	67.	d
32.	b	68.	a
33.	c	69.	d
34.	a	70.	b
35.	d	71.	b
36.	a	72.	a
37.	d	73.	b
38.	a	74.	a
39.	a	75.	a
40.	a	76.	a
41.	c	77.	b
42.	b	78.	c
43.	c	79.	a
44.	c	80.	d
45.	c	81.	c
46.	a	82.	d
47.	a	83.	a
48.	b	84.	d
49.	c	85.	d
50.	d	86.	a
51.	c	87.	a
52.	c	88.	d
53.	d	89.	d
54.	a	90.	b
55.	b	91.	b
56.	c	92.	b
57.	b	93.	d
58.	c	94.	a
59.	a	95.	a
60.	a	96.	c
61.	b	97.	b
62.	a	98.	b
63.	a	99.	a
64.	a	100.	a

Appendix 2

ANSWERS TO REVIEW STRIPS

CHAPTER 15

1. Rate: 60
   Rhythm: Regular
   P waves: 2 per QRS complex
   PRI: 0.16 second
   QRS: 0.04 second
   Interpretation: Second-degree heart block, Mobitz type II, 2:1 block

2. Rate: 30
   Rhythm: Regular
   P waves: Absent
   PRI: Absent
   QRS: 0.14 second
   Interpretation: Idioventricular rhythm

3. Rate: 90
   Rhythm: Irregular
   P waves: A
   PRI: A
   QRS: A
   Interpretation: Atrial fibrillation with unifocal PVCs

4. Rate: Ventricular 40; atrial 80
   Rhythm: Regular
   P waves: Present and upright
   PRI: Variable
   QRS: 0.10 second
   Interpretation: Third-degree (complete) heart block

5. Rate: 50
   Rhythm: Regular
   P waves: Inverted
   PRI: 0.08 second
   QRS: 0.04 second
   Interpretation: Junctional escape rhythm

6. Rate: 90
   Rhythm: Irregular
   P waves: A
   PRI: A
   Interpretation: Atrial fibrillation

7. Rate: 70
   Rhythm: Regular
   P waves: Present and upright
   PRI: 0.16 second
   QRS: 0.08 second
   Interpretation: Normal sinus rhythm (NSR)

8. Rate: 130
   Rhythm: Regular
   P waves: Present and upright
   PRI: 0.12 second
   QRS: 0.04 second
   Interpretation: Sinus tachycardia

9. Rate: 110
   Rhythm: Irregular (due to premature complexes)
   P waves: Present and upright
   PRI: 0.16 second
   QRS: 0.04 second (for normally conducted beats)
   Interpretation: Sinus rhythm with couplet PVCs

10. Rate: I
   Rhythm: I
   P waves: I
   PRI: I
   QRS: I
   Interpretation: Artifact

11. Rate: 70
   Rhythm: Irregular
   P waves: Present (for sinus complexes)
   PRI: 0.16 second
   QRS: 0.06 second (sinus complexes);
                0.14 second (PVCs)
   Interpretation: Sinus rhythm; unifocal premature ventricular complexes

12. Rate: 60
   Rhythm: Regular
   P waves: Present and upright
   PRI: 0.28 second
   QRS: 0.08 second
   Interpretation: Sinus rhythm with first-degree heart block

13. Rate: 70
   Rhythm: Regular
   P waves: I (flutter waves)
   PRI: I
   QRS: 0.04 second
   Interpretation: Atrial flutter

14. Rate: 70
    Rhythm: Paced rhythm
    P waves: A
    PRI: I
    QRS: 0.10 second
    Interpretation: Ventricular pacemaker

15. Rate: I
    Rhythm: I
    P waves: I
    PRI: I
    QRS: I
    Interpretation: Coarse ventricular fibrillation

16. Rate: 60
    Rhythm: Irregular (due to premature complexes)
    P waves: Present and upright (for sinus beats)
    PRI: 0.20 second
    QRS: 0.06 second
    Interpretation: Sinus rhythm with ventricular trigeminy

17. Rate: 50
    Rhythm: Atrial—regular; ventricular—regular
    P waves: Present and upright
    PRI: Variable
    QRS: 0.12 second
    Interpretation: Third-degree heart block (complete heart block)

18. Rate: 80
    Rhythm: Irregular (due to premature complexes)
    P waves: Present and upright (for sinus beats)
    PRI: 0.20 second
    QRS: 0.08 second (sinus beats)
    Interpretation: Sinus rhythm, with short run of ventricular tachycardia

19. Rate: 100
    Rhythm: Regular
    P waves: A
    PRI: I
    QRS: 0.12 second
    Interpretation: Accelerated idioventricular rhythm

20. Rate: 150
    Rhythm: Irregular
    P waves: Present and upright in first complex only; otherwise absent
    PRI: 0.12 second in first complex only; otherwise absent
    QRS: 0.06 second in first complex only; in other complexes, greater than 0.12 second
    Interpretation: Ventricular tachycardia

21. Rate: 60
    Rhythm: Atrial—regular; ventricular—regular
    P waves: Present and upright
    PRI: 0.16 second
    QRS: 0.04 second
    Interpretation: Normal sinus rhythm

22. Rate: 80
    Rhythm: Regular
    P waves: A
    PRI: I
    QRS: 0.04 second
    Interpretation: Accelerated junctional rhythm

23. Rate: 220
    Rhythm: Irregular
    P waves: I
    PRI: I
    QRS: Variable (0.12–0.24 second)
    Interpretation: Torsades de pointes

24. Rate: 180
    Rhythm: Regular
    P waves: Present and upright (in first 6 complexes)
    PRI: I (approximately 0.04 second)
    QRS: 0.04 second
    Interpretation: Supraventricular tachycardia

25. Rate: 80
    Rhythm: Irregular (due to premature complex)
    P waves: Present and upright (for sinus beats)
    PRI: 0.20 second
    QRS: 0.04 second
    Interpretation: Sinus rhythm with PACs (premature atrial complexes)

26. Rate: 90
    Rhythm: Regular
    P waves: Present and upright
    PRI: 0.16 second
    QRS: 0.08 second
    Interpretation: Normal sinus rhythm

27. Rate: 90
    Rhythm: Irregular
    P waves: Present and upright
    PRI: 0.16 second
    QRS: 0.04 second
    Interpretation: Sinus rhythm with PACs

28. Rate: 60
    Rhythm: Irregular
    P waves: Present and upright
    PRI: 0.16 second
    QRS: 0.04 second
    Interpretation: Sinus arrest

29. Rate: A
    Rhythm: A
    P waves: A
    PRI: A
    QRS: A
    Interpretation: Asystole

30. Rate: I
    Rhythm: I
    P waves: I
    PRI: I
    QRS: I
    Interpretation: Ventricular fibrillation (coarse)

31. Rate: 90
    Rhythm: Irregular (due to premature complexes)
    P waves: Present and upright for sinus beats
    PRI: 0.16 second
    QRS: 0.04 second
    Interpretation: Sinus rhythm with PACs (premature atrial complexes)

32. Rate: 120
    Rhythm: Regular
    P waves: Present; follow QRS complexes
    PRI: I
    QRS: 0.06 second
    Interpretation: Junctional tachycardia

33. Rate: 70
    Rhythm: Irregular
    P waves: Present and upright (for sinus beats)
    PRI: 0.12 second
    QRS: 0.04 second
    Interpretation: Sinus rhythm with ventricular trigeminy

34. Rate: 70
    Rhythm: Irregular
    P waves: Present and upright (for sinus beats)
    PRI: 0.16 second
    QRS: 0.04 second (sinus beats)
    Interpretation: Sinus rhythm with ventricular bigeminy

35. Rate: 80
    Rhythm: Atrial—regular; ventricular—regular
    P waves: Present and upright
    PRI: Variable
    QRS: 0.08 second
    Interpretation: Third-degree (complete) heart block

36. Rate: I
    Rhythm: Irregular
    P waves: A
    PRI: A
    QRS: I
    Interpretation: R on T phenomenon

37. Rate: 50
    Rhythm: Essentially regular
    P waves: Varying morphology
    PRI: 0.16 second
    QRS: 0.08 second
    Interpretation: Wandering atrial pacemaker (WAP)

38. Rate: 130
    Rhythm: Regular
    P waves: Present and upright
    PRI: 0.12 second
    QRS: 0.04 second
    Interpretation: Sinus tachycardia

39. Rate: A
    Rhythm: A
    P waves: A
    PRI: A
    QRS: A
    Interpretation: Ventricular fibrillation (shock delivered—end of strip)

40. Rate: 90
    Rhythm: Irregularly irregular
    P waves: A
    PRI: I
    QRS: 0.04 second
    Interpretation: Atrial fibrillation

41. Rate: 180
    Rhythm: Regular
    P waves: A
    PRI: A
    QRS: 0.16 second
    Interpretation: Ventricular tachycardia

42. Rate: 60
    Rhythm: Irregular (due to premature complexes)
    P waves: Present and upright (for sinus beats)
    PRI: 0.14 second
    QRS: 0.04 second
    Interpretation: Sinus rhythm with unifocal PVCs

43. Rate: 80
    Rhythm: Irregular (due to premature complex)
    P waves: A
    PRI: A
    QRS: 0.06 second
    Interpretation: Atrial fibrillation with 1 PAC

44. Rate: A
    Rhythm: I
    P waves: A
    PRI: A
    QRS: A
    Interpretation: Ventricular fibrillation

45. Rate: 100
    Rhythm: Regular
    P waves: Present and upright
    PRI: 0.16 second
    QRS: 0.08 second
    Interpretation: Sinus tachycardia with ST segment elevation

46. Rate: 40
    Rhythm: Regular
    P waves: Present and upright
    PRI: 0.16 second
    QRS: 0.04 second
    Interpretation: Sinus bradycardia

47. Rate: 120
    Rhythm: Regular
    P waves: Present and upright
    PRI: 0.18 second
    QRS: 0.04 second
    Interpretation: Sinus tachycardia

48. Rate: 40
    Rhythm: Irregular
    P waves: Present and upright
    PRI: Progressively prolonging
    QRS: 0.04 second
    Interpretation: Second-degree heart block, Mobitz type I, Wenchebach

49. Rate: Atrial—70; ventricular—40
   Rhythm: Atrial—regular; ventricular—regular
   P waves: Present and upright
   PRI: Variable
   QRS: 0.04 second
   Interpretation: Third-degree (complete) heart block

50. Rate: 40
   Rhythm: Regular
   P waves: A
   PRI: A
   QRS: 0.06 second
   Interpretation: Junctional escape rhythm

Glossary

A

absolute refractory period   stage of cell activity in which the cardiac cell cannot spontaneously depolarize

accelerated idioventricular rhythm (AIVR)   occurs when the rate of the ectopic pacemaker in an idioventricular rhythm exceeds 40 beats per minute

accelerated junctional rhythm   increased automaticity in the AV junction, causing the junction to discharge impulses at a rate faster than its intrinsic rate

accessory pathway   an irregular muscle connection between the atria and ventricles that bypasses the AV node

acetylcholine   the chemical neurotransmitter for the parasympathetic nervous system

acute myocardial infarction   (heart attack) results from a prolonged lack of blood flow to a portion of the myocardial tissue and results in a lack of oxygen

afterload   the resistance against which the heart must pump

agonal   when the rate of an IVR rhythm falls below 20 bpm, the rhythm may be called agonal

angina pectoris   pain that results from a reduction in blood supply to myocardial tissue

anion   an ion with a negative charge

aortic valve   the semilunar valve located between the left ventricle and the trunk of the aorta

arteries   thick-walled and muscular blood vessels that function under high pressure to convey blood from the heart out to the rest of the body

artifact   EKG waveforms from sources outside the heart

artificial pacemaker   a device that substitutes for the normal pacemaker cells of the heart's electrical conduction system

atherosclerosis   narrowed coronary arterial walls, secondary to fatty deposits

atrial dysrhythmias   the group of dysrhythmias produced when the SA node fails to generate an impulse and the atrial tissues or areas in the internodal pathways initiate an impulse

atrial fibrillation   when multiple disorganized ectopic atrial foci generate electrical activity at a very rapid rate (atrial rate varies from 350 to 750 bpm)

atrial flutter   when a single irritable site in the atria initiates many electrical impulses at a rapid rate, characterized by the presence of regular atrial activity with a picket-fence or sawtooth pattern

atrial kick   the final phase of diastole, atrial contraction forces remaining blood into the ventricles; provides 15–30% of ventricular filling

atrioventricular (AV) node   located on the floor of the right atrium near the opening of the coronary sinus and just above the tricuspid valve; at the level of the AV node, the electrical activity is delayed approximately 0.05 second

atrium   upper chamber of the heart

automaticity   the ability of cardiac pacemaker cells to generate their own electrical impulses spontaneously without external (or nervous) stimulation

autonomic nervous system   regulates functions of the body that are involuntary, or not under conscious control

AV junction   the region where the AV node joins the bundle of His

B

Bachmann's bundle   a subdivision of the anterior internodal tract, conducts electrical activity from the SA node to the left atrium

baseline   the straight line seen on an EKG strip; it represents the beginning and end point of all waves

Beck's triad   muffled heart sounds, JVD, and narrowing pulse pressure

bipolar leads   have one positive electrode and one negative electrode

bradycardia   heart rate of less than 60 bpm

bundle branches   two main branches, the right bundle branch and the left bundle branch, conduct electrical activity from the bundle of His down to the Purkinje network

bundle of His   the conduction pathway that leads out of the AV node and is also traditionally referred to as the *common bundle*

C

capillaries   tiny blood vessels that allow for the exchange of oxygen, nutrients, and waste products between the blood and body tissues; "connectors" between arteries and veins

capture   noted by the presence of a spike and wide QRS complexes, the presence of an adequate carotid pulse and blood pressure, and an increased level of consciousness

cardiac cycle   the actual time sequence between ventricular contraction and ventricular relaxation

cardiac output   the amount of blood pumped by the left ventricle in 1 minute

cardiac tamponade   an excess accumulation of fluid in the pericardial sac

cardiogenic shock   when left ventricular function is so severely compromised that the heart can no longer meet the metabolic requirements of the body

cation   an ion with a positive charge

chest pain   is the most common presenting symptom of cardiac disease, as well as the most common complaint by patients

chordae tendineae   fine chords of dense connective tissue that attach to papillary muscles in the wall of the ventricles

circulation   movement through a course (the body) which leads back to the initial point (the heart)

compensatory pause   a pause that occurs after an ectopic beat in which the SA node is unaffected and the cadence of the heart is uninterrupted

conductivity   the ability of cardiac cells to receive an electrical stimulus and then transmit it to other cardiac cells

congestive heart failure   when the heart's stroke volume becomes severely diminished and causes an overload of fluid in systemic tissues

contractility   also referred to as rhythmicity, is the ability of cardiac cells to shorten and cause cardiac muscle contraction in response to an electrical stimulus

D

demand or synchronous pacemaker   generates electrical impulses when the patient's heart rate falls below a predetermined rate

diaphoresis   profuse sweating

diastole   is synonymous with ventricular relaxation

dyspnea   labored breathing

dysrhythmia   abnormal heart rhythm

E

EKG waveforms   a wave or waveform recorded on an EKG strip refers to movement away from the baseline or isoelectric line and is represented as a positive deflection (above the isoelectric line) or as a negative deflection (below the isoelectric line)

electrocardiogram   graphic representation of the electrical activity of the heart

electrocardiograph   machine used to record the electrocardiogram

electrode   an adhesive pad that contains conductive gel and is designed to be attached to the patient's skin

electrolyte   a substance or compound whose molecules dissociate into charged components, or ions, when placed in water, producing positively and negatively charged ions

endocardium   the innermost layer of the heart; composed of thin connective tissue

epicardium   the smooth outer surface of the heart

excitability   the ability of cardiac cells to respond to an electrical stimulus, a characteristic shared by all cardiac cells

F

first-degree heart block   the most usual form of block, results from excessive conduction delay in the AV node

fixed-rate or asynchronous pacemaker   programmed to deliver electrical impulses at a constant selected rate

G

generator   controls the rate and strength of each electrical impulse

H

heart blocks   electrical conduction system disorders

heart failure   the inability of the myocardium to meet the cardiac output demands of the body

heart rate   the number of contractions, or beats, per minute of the heart

heart rhythm   the sequential beating of the heart as a result of the generation of electrical impulses

hemodynamically stable   refers to a patient who presents with a normal blood pressure (normotensive), absence of chest pain, and no notable change in mental status

hemodynamically unstable   refers to a patient who presents with hypotension (low blood pressure), chest pain, shortness of breath, and changes in mental status

hypovolemia   decreased blood volume

hypoxia   low oxygen level

I

idioventricular rhythms (IVRs)   (also called ventricular escape rhythms) result when the discharge rate of higher pacemakers become less than that of the ventricles or when impulses from higher pacemakers fail to reach the ventricles

inferior vena cava   collects blood from the rest of the body

internodal tracts   distribute the electrical impulse throughout the atria and transmit the impulse from the SA node to the AV node

interpolated beat   occurs when a PVC falls between two sinus beats without interfering with the rhythm

J

J point   the point where the QRS complex meets the ST segment

junctional escape rhythm   when the SA node fails to generate an impulse or if the rate of impulse generation falls below that of the AV node, then the AV node will assume the role of the pacemaker; the resulting rhythm is called a junctional escape rhythm

junctional rhythms   rhythms that are initiated in the area of the AV junction

junctional tachycardia rhythm   a rhythm arising from the AV junctional tissue at a rate of 100–180 bpm

junctional tachycardia   when the junctional firing rate exceeds 100 bpm

L

lead a pair of electrodes such as chest Lead I, II, MCL

lead wires relay the electrical impulse from the generator to the myocardium

leads electrodes connected to the monitor or EKG machine by wires

left ventricular failure when a patient's left ventricle ceases to function in an adequate capacity as to sustain sufficient systemic cardiac output

M

mediastinum the central section of the thorax (chest cavity)

mitral (or bicuspid) valve similar in structure to the tricuspid valve but has only two cusps and is located between the left atrium and the left ventricle

morphology shape of the PVC

multifocal PVCs with different shapes that originate from different sites within the ventricles

multifocal atrial tachycardia (MAT) the rhythm created when the rate of the wandering atrial pacemaker rhythm reaches 100 beats per minute (bpm) or greater

myocardial ischemia decreased supply of oxygenated blood to the heart

myocardial working cells responsible for generating the physical contraction of the heart muscle

myocardium the thick middle layer of the heart composed primarily of cardiac muscle cells and responsible for the heart's ability to contract

N

neuropathy inability to perceive pain due to diseases of the nerves

nitroglycerin causes dilation of the blood vessels that consequently reduces the workload of the heart

noncompensatory pause the pause that occurs after an ectopic beat, when the SA node is depolarized

nonsustained rhythm a run of VT that lasts for less than 30 seconds

norepinephrine the chemical neurotransmitter for the sympathetic nervous system

normal sinus rhythm the rhythm that occurs when the SA node has generated an impulse that followed the normal pathway of the electrical conduction system and led to atrial and ventricular depolarization

O

oxygen the most important drug that any patient with chest pain can receive

P

P wave represents depolarization of the left and right atria

pacemaker spike the EKG wave produced by an artificial pacemaker

palpitations a sensation that the heart is skipping beats and/or beating rapidly

parasympathetic nervous system regulates the calmer ("rest and digest") functions

paroxysmal refers to a sudden onset or cessation or both

paroxysmal junctional tachycardia (PJT) rhythm a junctional tachycardia rhythm that is observed to begin or end abruptly

paroxysmal rhythm a rhythm observed to start or end abruptly

pericarditis an inflammation of the serous pericardium

pericardium closed, two-layered sac that surrounds the heart; "potential space" between the visceral and parietal layers of the pericardium holds a small amount of pericardial fluid (approximately 10–20 cc)

peripheral vascular resistance (PVR) the amount of opposition to blood flow offered by the arterioles

permanent pacemakers implanted inside the patient's upper left chest (most commonly) and are left in place

PR interval measures the time intervals from the onset of atrial contraction to the onset of ventricular contraction

preload the pressure in the ventricles at the end of diastole

premature atrial contraction (PAC) a single, electrical impulse that originates outside the SA node in the atria

premature junctional contractions (PJCs) initiate from a single site in the AV junction and arise earlier than the next anticipated complex of the underlying rhythm

premature ventricular complex a single, ectopic (out-of-place) complex that occurs earlier than the next expected complex and arises from an irritable site in the ventricles

Prinzmetal's angina or vasospastic angina form of angina that can occur when the coronary arteries experience spasms and constrict

pulmonary circulation when blood leaves the heart through the right ventricle and travels into the pulmonary artery to the lungs and back through the pulmonary veins to the left atrium

pulmonary edema backup of blood in the pulmonary system that causes plasma to mix with and displace alveolar air

pulmonic valve the semilunar valve located between the right ventricle and the pulmonary artery

pulseless electrical activity (PEA) the absence of a palpable pulse and myocardial muscle activity with the presence of organized electrical activity (excluding VT or VF) on the cardiac monitor

pulsus paradoxus evidenced by a systolic blood pressure that drops more than 10–15 mmHg during inspiration

Purkinje's Network a network of fibers that carries electrical impulses directly to ventricular muscle cells

Q

QRS complex consists of the Q, R, and S waves and represents the conduction of the electrical impulse from the bundle of His throughout the ventricular muscle, or ventricular depolarization

R

rapid ventricular response a ventricular rate of 100–150 bpm

reentry the reactivation of myocardial tissue for a second or subsequent time by the same electrical impulse

relative refractory period the period when repolarization is almost complete, and the cardiac cell can be stimulated to contract prematurely if the stimulus is much stronger than normal

rhythm strip or EKG strip the printed record of the electrical activity of the heart

right heart failure when the right ventricle ceases to function properly, causing an increase in pressure within the right atrium, thus forcing the blood backward into the systemic venous system

S

SA node commonly referred to as the primary pacemaker of the heart because it normally depolarizes more rapidly than any other part of the conduction system

salvos another name given to a run or grouping of 3 or more PVCs in a row

second-degree AV block, Mobitz type I, or Wenckenbach the progressive prolongation of the electrical impulse delay at the AV node produces an increase in the length of the PR interval

second-degree AV block, or Mobitz type II a more serious dysrhythmia that occurs when there is an intermittent interruption in the electrical conduction system near or below the AV junction

semilunar valves　serve to prevent the backflow of blood into the ventricles and each valve contains three semilunar (or moon-shaped) cusps

sensing　is simply the capability of a pacemaker to recognize inherent electrical conduction system activity

sinus arrest rhythm　When the sinus node fails to discharge, the absence of a PQRST interval is noted on the rhythm strip

sinus bradycardia　in this rhythm, the SA node discharges impulses at a rate of less than 60 beats per minute

sinus dysrhythmia　an irregular rhythm produced when the P-to-P intervals and the R-to-R intervals change with respirations

sinus tachycardia　a variant of normal sinus rhythm; the rate is generally considered to be 100–160 beats per minute

site of origin　rhythms are classified according to the heart structure or structures in which they begin

slow ventricular response　a ventricular rate of less than 60 bpm

specialized group　responsible for controlling the rate and rhythm of the heart by coordinating regular depolarization and are found in the electrical conduction system of the heart

ST segment　begins with the end of the QRS complex and ends with the onset of the T wave

"stable" or predictable angina　a particular activity may elicit chest pain

Starling's law of the heart　the more the myocardial fibers are stretched, up to a certain point, the more forceful the subsequent contraction will be

stroke volume　the volume of blood pumped out of one ventricle of the heart in a single beat or contraction

superior vena cava　drains blood from the head and neck

supraventricular　above the ventricles

supraventricular tachycardia (SVT)　a general term that encompasses all fast (tachy-) dysrhythmias in which the heart rate is greater than 100 bpm

sustained rhythm　a rhythm that lasts for more than 30 seconds

sympathetic nervous system　responsible for preparation of the body for physical activity ("fight or flight")

systemic circulation　the circulation of blood as it leaves the left ventricle and travels through the arteries, capillaries, and veins of the entire body system and back to the primary receptacle of the heart (the right atrium)

systole or ventricular systole　is consistent with the simultaneous contraction of the ventricles

T

T wave　produced by ventricular repolarization or relaxation; represents ventricular repolarization and follows the ST segment

tachycardia　heart rate greater than 100 bpm

temporary pacemakers　used to sustain a patient's heart rate in emergent situations

third-degree AV block (complete)　the most serious type of heart block; the atria and ventricles are completely blocked or separated from each other electrically at or below the AV node; ventricular rate will most commonly be between 20 and 40 bpm

threshold　refers to the point at which a stimulus will produce a cell response

thrombus formation　the most common cause of myocardial infarction; results in blockage of the coronary artery

torsades de pointes　similar to ventricular tachycardia; morphology of QRS complexes show variations in width and shape; life-threatening dysrhythmia

transcutaneous pacing (TCP)　commonly called external cardiac pacing, consists of two large electrode pads, which are most commonly placed in an anterior-posterior position on the patient's chest to condcut electrical impulses through the skin to the heart

transvenous pacing　(through a vein) a lead wire is inserted through the skin and threaded into a large vein leading into the right side of the heart and controlled by an external power source

tricuspid valve   named for its three cusps; located between the right atrium and the right ventricle

U

unifocal   PVCs that are alike in appearance

unstable angina   pain not elicited by activity that most commonly occurs while the patient is at rest; also referred to as "preinfarctional" angina

V

vagal maneuvers   methods utilized to stimulate baroreceptors (located in the internal carotid and aortic arch); when these receptors are stimulated, the vagus nerves release acetylcholine, resulting in a slowing of the heart rate

veins   blood vessels that carry blood back to the heart, operate under low pressure, and are relatively thin-walled

ventricle   lower chamber of the heart

ventricular asystole   the absence of all ventricular activity; also called cardiac standstill or asystole; the absence of all cardiac electrical activity

ventricular fibrillation (V fib, VF)   is a fatal dysrhythmia that occurs as a result of multiple weak ectopic foci in the ventricles; there is no coordinated atrial or ventricular contraction and no palpable pulse

ventricular tachycardia (VT or V tach)   rhythm in which three or more PVCs arise in sequence at a rate of greater than 100 beats per minute; commonly overrides the normal pacemaker of the heart

W

wandering atrial pacemaker (WAP) rhythms   occur when pacemaker sites wander, or travel, from the SA node to other pacemaker sites in the atria, the internodal pathways, or the AV node

Wolff-Parkinson-White syndrome (WPW)   preexcitation syndrome and atrioventricular conduction disorder characterized by two AV conduction pathways and is often identified by a characteristic delta wave seen on an electrocardiogram at the beginning of the QRS complex

Index

Croydon Health Sciences Library
Mayday University Hospital
London Road
Thornton Heath
Surrey CR7 7YE